The Gift of Care

The Gift of Care

2nd edition

HARRY VAN BOMMEL

Resources Supporting Family
& Community Legacies Inc.
Toronto 2013

Cover illustration by Diane Huson

Library and Archives Canada Cataloguing in Publication

van Bommel, Harry
The gift of care / Harry van Bommel. -- 2nd ed.
Includes bibliographical references and index.
ISBN 978-1-55307-070-2
1. Hospice care. 2. Palliative treatment. I. Resources Supporting Family and Community Legacies Inc. II. Title.

RT87.T45V33 2013 616.02'9 C2012-908424-7

Made possible through the generous contributions of:

Salem Alaton, Diane Bolduc, Carol Brock, Jeanette Browne, Heather Campbell, Rubin Cohen, Judith Cox, Sonja & Lynn Davie, Hung Der, Jutta & John Genova, Heather Gollob, Diane and Bill Huson, Anne & Alvin Isenberg, Louise LeBlanc, Michael & Patricia Man, T.D. Man, Eileen McArthur, Sandra McBay, Ann McClean-Gatto, Josi Perotto, Albert Pinhas, Jacquelyn Saad, Irene Sakata, Stan Salsberg, Deb Thivierge and Dena Maule and Belinda Marchese of Hospice Toronto for their help in this project .

Resources Supporting Family and Community Legacies Inc.
11 Miniot Circle
Toronto, ON
Canada M1K 2K1\
(416) 264-4665
e-mail: harry@legacies.ca
web site: www.legacies.ca
bookstore: www.legacies-inc.ca

Contents

This book is dedicated:

in gratitude to my parents, grandfather and all those who have allowed me the gift of caring for them,

in honour of the thousands who have taken part in my caregiving workshops and presentations so they could learn and share their own experiences with all of us,

with respect to Jane and Matthew Pearson who teach us as much as they learn,

and with pride and love to Janet, Joanna and Bram.

Acknowledgements

This book is based on workshops that I present to **professional** and **volunteer** health care providers, **families** and **patients**. I am very grateful to the thousands of participants who have shared their experiences with each other and with me during these workshops. I am also grateful to those who have made suggestions of how I could improve the workshops and make them even more practical.

I am also grateful to the many professionals and volunteers in both health care and hospice palliative care who have reviewed my other publications over the years to help ensure that they are as helpful and accurate as possible.

A special thank you to **Jeanette Browne** who was the Volunteer Co-ordinator at Hospice

Toronto and has worked in the hospice field in various capacities since the 1990s. She was the first Education Coordinator at the Community Hospice Association of Ontario and, therefore, helped many community hospices develop their initial programs for staff and volunteers. Her expertise in this field and other community service organizations helps ensure that the information in this book continues to help a wide range of professionals and volunteers as they provide the gift of care.

I would like to thank my wife, **Janet Klees**, for editing the first draft of this book (as she does all my books!) and for her support and encouragement of the work I do. Writing can be a time consuming task and she always gladly frees up my time so that I can work when I need to. Also, to our children, **Joanna** and **Bram**, for their enthusiasm and pride in what I do. One cannot work in this field without recognizing the gifts of support received from family and friends. It means more to me than they might suspect and I am grateful.

I gratefully acknowledge that funding for this book was made possible by the generous contributions of: Salem Alaton, Diane Bolduc,

Carol Brock, Jeanette Browne, Heather Campbell, Rubin Cohen, Judith Cox, Sonja & Lynn Davie, Hung Der, Jutta & John Genova, Heather Gollob, Diane and Bill Huson, Anne & Alvin Isenberg, Louise LeBlanc, Michael & Patricia Man, T.D. Man, Eileen McArthur, Sandra McBay, Ann McClean-Gatto, Josi Perotto, Albert Pinhas, Jacquelyn Saad, Irene Sakata, Stan Salsberg, Deb Thivierge and Dena Maule and Belinda Marchese of Hospice Toronto for their help in this project.

A Note on Language

I will use several terms throughout this book. Health care vocabulary changes so often it is hard to keep up. For consistency I have used the following terms:

Patient is the person receiving care. In many programs this person is also called client, consumer, decision-maker or resident. Patient, however, is the term used most often and is, therefore, not confused with clients who may include the patient's primary caregiver or family member.

Hospice palliative care means care given to someone facing their final illness. When Dr. Balfour Mount coined the phrase "palliative care" in the mid 1970s, it was used in Canada rather than "hospice care" as it was called in Britain where it was founded by Dr. Cicely Saunders in the 1960s.

He chose "palliative care" because "hospice" translated into French could mean a poor house where people go to die. He wanted a term that was more easily translated in both English and French – palliative care or *soins palliatifs*.

Sadly, we have confused an often-confusing term by combining them into "hospice palliative care." However, we are stuck with this new term and so I use it here. I sometimes use the shorter version of "hospice care" or "palliative care" because they are actually quite interchangeable grammatically. What has changed is that hospice care now often refers to care given in the community and palliative care is that which is given by physicians in hospital-based programs.

Care providers are health care professionals and volunteers.

Family members or **family caregivers** may provide care but their principal role must remain that of spouse, child, parent, closest friends, or grandparent. They must never be seen nor labeled as only 'caregivers.' Family is defined as those people the person identifies as family and often includes their best friends.

Volunteers refer to those caregivers who volunteer their help through a formal program or agency such as a community hospice service or hospital volunteer department.

Introduction

To care FOR someone,
you must care ABOUT them.

This book is meant to provide practical information, support and encouragement to all those who provide care – **family caregivers, friends, professional and volunteer providers**. Sometimes examples apply to all caregivers while other examples may be specific to volunteers or family members.

Although this book is primarily about providing hospice palliative care, I hope that professionals and volunteers in other fields of health care will learn from this ancient philosophy of care. It is highly compatible with modern health care when the two are combined and the patient and family are truly treated as the prime decision makers and recipients of care.

This book is partly based on the care I provided my mother, my grandfather and then my father when they were living at home until they died. I cared for them in their homes and these experiences were life defining and life affirming for each of us. I learned to be a better son, better spouse, better friend, better parent and a better neighbor.

Part of the information is also based on the hospital birth of our son and home birth of our daughter plus the home care I have been privileged to provide to family and friends recovering from surgery, injury or illness.

Providing care is different from receiving it. I learned this when I was on the receiving end of care after various illnesses and surgeries. It is receiving care that taught me that **the gift of care must be mutually beneficial to be truly a gift.**

This book contains original material not found in any of my other publications. It is based on the workshops I provide to health care and hospice palliative care professionals, volunteers and families. Many of them have asked that I write a short book expanding on the ideas I present in my workshops.

The times family members spend caring for their loved ones are times filled with a roller coaster of emotions from their highest highs to their lowest lows. For most of us family members, there is no road map so we stumble along together. I hope that this book provides you with the knowledge you need and an acknowledgement of what you do well so that you can help other people on a similar roller coaster ride.

When you provide care to people like me, you have an opportunity to ensure that your patients' and their families' last months together are filled with the type of caring we hope to have in our own last months. ***Every day you have an opportunity to make that dramatic difference in someone's life. Every day!***

And everyday, that difference you make enhances your life in immeasurable ways. This is a mutual gift. You will give your knowledge, skills and compassion and you will receive some of the same in return. Sometimes you will give more and other times you will receive more. That is part of the gift of what you do.

Use this gift well. No other experiences in life

are filled with as much potential. You are part of a time-limited yet opportunity-rich set of experiences.

Local examples of this type of care are provided in your community by people who have gone through these experiences themselves and by hospice palliative care programs, visiting home nurses, knowledgeable family physicians who make house calls, pharmacists who provide advice, funeral directors who provide information and so many others. Find them, learn from them, observe them and treasure them all.

Traditional hospice palliative care is the model all health care providers (professionals and volunteers) need to apply to their work. Whether you work in acute care, long-term care, respite care, community health and related fields, the hospice palliative care model combines ancient wisdom with modern health care.

Health care is providing excellent physical, emotional, spiritual, and information supports to patients and their loved ones from conception to death and bereavement.

Hospice palliative care is providing excellent physical, emotional, spiritual, and information supports to patients and their loved ones in the last period of life.

If health care met people's needs, hospice palliative care would not be necessary. Since much of modern health care does not meet dying patients' needs, hospice palliative care should be brought in as soon as possible to help people in their last period of living.

This point is crucial to your understanding of the rest of this book. If health care met people's needs, hospice palliative care would not be necessary. We would not need a separate program to meet people's needs because health care providers would already be trained and experienced in meeting people's physical, emotional, spiritual and information needs. **Therefore, hospice palliative care should never try to emulate the systemic approach to care that exists in present-day hospitals and long-term care facilities.** Rather, it should become the model that others copy to enhance their care at all points of a person's life. People should not have to be dying to get excellent physical, emotional, spiritual and informational care.

Look at your own life and work. Ask yourself the following questions.

1. Have you ever been patient? Would you like to be a patient again? Why or why not?
2. Have you ever received home care before? Was it enough? Why or why not?
3. Would you, as a health care professional or volunteer, recommend your work to your children as a career? Why or why not?
4. Do you look forward to receiving the service you provide now to others and in the settings where you provide that service? Why or why not?

Ask yourself how patients in your care have similar needs to all of us and identify how you can meet those needs even more than you do now.

A chronic care patient spoke the patient perspective that best summarizes what care providers need to understand about care:

I have been chronically ill for twelve years. Stroke. Paralysis. That's what I'm dealing with now. I've

gone to rehab program after rehab program. I may be one of the most rehabilitated people on the face of the earth. I should be President. I've worked with a lot of people, and I've seen many types and attitudes. People try very hard to help me do my best on my own. They understand the importance of that self-sufficiency, and so do I. They're positive and optimistic. I admire them for their perseverance. My body is broken, but they still work very hard with it. They're very dedicated. I having nothing but respect for them. But I must say this: I have never, ever, met someone who sees me as a whole… Can you understand this? Can you? No one sees me and helps me see myself as being complete, as is. No one really sees how that's true, at the deepest level. Everything else is Band-Aids, you know.
[Ram Dass & Paul Gorman in *How Can I Help?*]

Seeing someone as a whole is our greatest gift to each other. When you look at yourself in the mirror, do you see the person you feel like "inside?" Are you sometimes surprised by how you look? Most of us do not feel how we look. We often feel younger than we look. I certainly am thinner in my mind than in the mirror!

When my grandfather was dying, he was 92 years old. I asked him one day what he missed most in his life. After several quiet minutes he answered: "I miss my mother." She had been dead for 53 years. He had a wife, 10 children and 35 grandchildren but he still missed his mother most. That was a very telling moment for me. It reminded me that someone who is "old," a recipient of The Netherlands highest civilian honor, a successful businessman and so much more still had elements of his youth inside him. When he looked in the mirror, he saw an old man yet his heart and mind had many elements left of his childhood. In hindsight, that is not a surprise but at the time (I was 25 when I asked him the question) it was a revelation.

Mr. G.[1] was a 70-year old man with a cancer that ate away his nose and mouth leaving an ugly tumor in their place. He wanted to die. His wife agreed he should die. He was not in pain. He was well loved by his family and friends. His spiritual community was very supportive. But he could not

---

1 van Bommel, Harry. (2002). *Family hospice care.*, pages 24-25.

deal with the constant emotional pain of watching people's faces as they looked at his tumor. Inside he was the man he always was but in the mirror he was horribly disfigured and it pained him to watch people look at him.

The palliative care team caring for him at Parkwood Hospital in London, Ontario had real questions about their own beliefs of caring for this man at the end of life. Never in their experience has someone challenged their views on euthanasia as profoundly. They could all easily imagine themselves in his place and understand his request to die to avoid the terrible trauma of people's responses to how he looked.

Mr. G had a 6-year old granddaughter who desperately wanted to see her Grandpa. Her mother (Mr G's daughter) did not want her to see her grandfather like that. Mr. G did not want to see her either and the palliative care team at the hospital thought it best she not see him.

However, like so many 6-year girls and boys, when they really want something they pester and hound their parents until they get their way. Finally, the parents and grandparents and palliative care team all agreed she could visit on the condition that the team prepare her before she went into the room.

As only a 6-year old can do, she sat in her chair with an air of complete indifference listening to their chatter until she was finally told she could go and visit her grandfather. She ran from the room down the hall to his hospital room, rushed through the door and up to his bed and encircled his neck with a great big hug. She said, "I love you Grandpa. Please don't go."

This little girl reminded her parents, grandparents and palliative care team to see her Grandpa as a whole man and how to nurture that caring spirit. She saw the whole man within the body rather than the tumor on his face. She reminded her grandfather to look within his heart rather than to look in the mirror. She gave him the gift of life when others were wondering if the gift of death might not be easier for him. She reminded him that he was still a grandfather and not just a patient. His 'work' was not done – she still needed him.

In a lighter vein, she may have been a Star Trek fan where characters with 'ugly' faces become characters we become interested in. We cheer for them when good things happen to them during the show and even grieve a little when bad things happen to them. Some fans grow fond of the character regardless of how they look. Their makeup is often 'disfiguring' (e.g., Klingons) and not very attractive the first time we see it, yet fans grow accustomed to it and find the person inside the costume physically attractive at some level.

Part of our inherent nurturing spirit comes from our own belief systems. Dr. Dorothy C.H. Ley was a founder of the hospice movement in Canada. A hematologist for most of her professional life she saw so many patients die from their cancer and decided that a better way must be found. In her subsequent palliative care work she concluded that effective care required meeting people's physical, emotional, spiritual and information needs. However, it was the spiritual aspects of care that provided "the heart of hospice."

> *Spiritual care lies at the heart of hospice. It says we are here. We will be with you in your living and your dying. We will free you from pain and*

> *give you the freedom to find your own meaning in your own life – your way. We will comfort you and those you love – not always with words, often with a touch or a glance. We will bring you hope – not for tomorrow but for this day.We will not leave you. We will watch with you.We will be there.*[2]

Spirituality as to do with who we are as people. Religion has to do with how we practice our spirituality, if at all, through various religious beliefs, practices and rituals. We are all spiritual people in the sense that we all have a need to know our lives have value and meaning. We are all children of God, however we describe God, and we are connected to each other, and to all nature, as members of a living community.

The only thing that separates us spiritually is our belief that separateness is possible. Our spirituality is often best expressed in times of great joy or distress.

Lyn Zimbler, a South African woman living with multiple sclerosis, wrote a book about her

---

2 Ley, Dorothy C.H. (1994). *The heart of hospice.* dedication page.

journey with this condition. She concluded that:

> *It seems to me that the gift hidden under the wings of this monstrously demanding dragon, is the gift of a wiser love and a more humble understanding.*[3]

It is in this spirit of a wiser love and a more humble understanding that this book is dedicated to all of of us who provide and receive care so that we can, together, meet the physical, emotional, spiritual and information needs of those living through their final illness.

---

3 Personal correspondence with the South African writer

CHAPTER 1

Understand Basic Home and Hospice Care

This book is primarily about hospice palliative care. That said, most of the principles and tips provided throughout the book also apply to home care situations when you are caring for someone who has had a baby, is recovering from surgery or an illness, or who has a condition that requires long-term care at home.

This book is based on the assumption that we can choose how we cope with our own illness or that of someone else.

Any time you provide care to someone else, you have an incredible opportunity to slow down your life and remind yourself that nurturing relationships is the single greatest key to our personal and professional happiness.

HOSPICE PALLIATIVE CARE

Hospice palliative care is about trying to meet a person's physical, emotional, spiritual and information needs. It is best practiced in a person's own home. When that is not possible it can and must be practiced as best as possible within other settings such as:

- the home of a family member or friend of the patient
- a free-standing hospice
- within a long-term care facility (including nursing homes) and within hospitals.

PAIN AND SYMPTOM CONTROL

Most people can be relatively pain free, comfortable and alert until they die. The days of people shouting out to die because the pain hurts so badly can be over for each patient who receives excellent hospice palliative care whether formally through a program or informally through physicians who are trained in pain and symptom control.

If a patient is suffering severe pain, get the doctor in charge to check with a palliative care specialist who can suggest methods to reduce the pain now. We have all the knowledge and skills, right now, to manage overwhelming pain. All of the pain may not go away. Most of us suffer from some physical pain from aging, arthritis, back problems, etc. However, unbearable pain is never necessary.

The secret to effective pain control (relief) is giving the **right drug(s)**, in the **right amount**, in the **right way** and at the **right time**. This balance requires physicians and other hospice team members to do proper, ongoing assessments of a person's pain and to consult with others who may have information that is helpful. Proper pain medication usually prevents overwhelming pain from returning while keeping the patient alert. If pain does suddenly increase (called 'breakthrough pain') extra medication must be immediately available to relieve it. In those rare cases when pain cannot be relieved enough, a person can be placed in a drug-induced coma for a period of time to alleviate the pain. No one needs to suffer the type of unmanaged pain that many of us have witnessed our parents and grandparents suffer.

Once pain is managed, other symptoms like

vomiting, bedsores, and dry mouths are more easily controlled.

Remember that other medical and complementary therapies can reduce pain and symptoms. Use those that are most helpful and proven in the circumstances.

PERSONALITY

People's basic personalities do not change when they find out they have a terminal or life-threatening illness or when they are grieving. How they dealt with stressful or traumatic situations in the past is likely how they cope now.

YOUR ROLE

Caring for others in such a personal and intimate way is one of the most fulfilling and life-defining opportunities in our lives. When you care for someone else you know in your heart, mind and soul that you are making a real difference in that person's life. Caregiving gives us that unique opportunity to remember what is truly valuable in our lives and within our families and community. Caring is not always easy. It can be physically exhausting, mentally taxing and emotionally draining. It can also be exhilarating, rejuvenating, peaceful, joyful and awe inspiring.

Choose a role that is comfortable and supportive to the person who is dying and to those who are grieving. You should also get the support from family and friends you need to continue to help others. Hospice care is about mutually caring for each other.

Not everyone you care for will be gentle, kind, grateful or thoughtful. Some have life experiences that preclude them from having such characteristics – especially as they near the end of their lives.

Everyone, however, deserves the best care you can give them. That said, it does not mean you have to accept abuse or continuing unkindness. You are allowed to ask people to be civil and respectful. Just because someone is dying does not mean their community and family roles stop. They should still be expected to follow the general principles of a reasonable civil and respectful behavior. If they cannot behave that way to you, you can ask someone else with whom the patient is more comfortable to provide more of the care. If the patient is unkind and abusive to everyone, then someone in authority (family member, physician, nurse or administrator) needs to lay down the rules more forcefully.

CHAPTER 2

Basic Assumptions

There are a number of basic assumptions that can help you make ethical decisions in how you work. Many of you will have these basic assumptions already. They are probably part of why you instinctively do some things very well. By identifying these assumptions, and becoming more conscious of them, you are more likely to use them all the time. When instincts become part of your conscious thinking, they also become part of the discussions you will have with other care providers. You will be better able to explain why you do certain things or why you talk in a certain way with people and about the people for whom you care.

RELATIONSHIPS

Relationships are more important than things, work or even good health. So often we talk about the importance of relationships in our lives and then ignore the most important relationships we actually have. Rather than nurture our relationships with our spouse, children, parents, grandparents, extended family and our best friends we actually end up spending more time with our work colleagues, the people who attend the same recreation centre, faith community or strangers at the local pub.

If we are going to provide the best care possible to those going through their last illness and to their families, we need to model what we preach about the importance of relationships. We need to nurture those we love most. We need to recognize that things, work or good health are not more important. Our work needs priority when we are working but our relationships need priority when we are not working.

An example of why even good health cannot take precedence over the importance of relationships is the story of "Liam" (name changed). Liam was a man in his 30s who was in one of my palliative care courses at a community college. He heard that my wife was pregnant and he knew that we already had a son. He congratulated me on the news of the pregnancy and then he said, "I bet you are praying for a girl now eh?"

I replied, "No, we are just praying for a baby." He nodded and pretended to hit the side of his head. "Of course, that was not very politically correct of me was it? You are not supposed to wish that someone gets a girl or boy. But I bet you are praying for a healthy baby."

Again I replied, "No, we are just praying for a baby."

Liam was confused. "I'm sorry I don't get it. I understand it is not correct to say you want a boy or a girl but everyone wants a healthy baby!"

"If we prayed for a 'healthy' baby and our baby was born unhealthy in some way, what would be our first response? What would be the first response of our family and the care providers in the room? We don't want the first response to be one of sadness, pity or even shock. We want our baby to be alive and welcomed with all the excitement and joy that every baby should experience upon their birth."

I was not trying to tell this man that we wanted an unhealthy baby to prove we are lovely people. I was trying to help him understand that the relationship between parent and child should not be based on whether the baby is healthy or not. Our bond is based on loving parents nurturing their baby.

At the other end of life, the assumption must be the same. We nurture and care for those we love regardless of their wealth, health or their accomplishments. Those that we care for professionally or as volunteers deserve to be seen in the most positive light with our first priority to help them nurture the relationships that are most important in their lives. We should not try to become another important relationship as much as to help nurture the existing ones.

You can nurture and care for others using this assumption about the fundamental importance of nurturing relationships. Here are the top 10 ways how.

1. Recognize that you are directly connected to everyone you meet; even people you do not like. We are all members of the human family. Although you are a care provider now, one day you will be the recipient of care.

2. Although no one can like everyone, everyone can be treated with respect, compassion (walking with a person through this period in their lives), excellent medical and palliative care and spiritual love.
3. Whatever draws people to you personally and professionally are exactly the skills you need to use when helping someone in their final months and days. If you are a great listener, then the person will probably want to talk to you. If you are a jokester, then the person will benefit from your sense of humor and 'weird' perspectives on life and death. If you are a 'do-er,' then they may turn to you to help with the practical legal, financial and funeral preparations. If you are a nurturer, they may ask you to help them care for their family after they have died. Whatever draws people to you is what you can best use to help someone. Although a hospice palliative care course can help professionals and volunteers expand their skills base, for family and friends, they really need to concentrate on what they already do very well. They should never feel like they need to read

a ton of books or take courses to help a loved one live fully until they die.

4. Friends are not paid, therefore, staff cannot be true friends. They can always be friendly, supportive, encouraging and excellent listeners, but they cannot be true friends unless they also spend lots of their free time with the person, invite them over for special holidays and celebrations, or have their family join your family for activities. What you can always do is help nurture and encourage the natural relationships people already have with their family, friends, neighbors and acquaintances.
5. Some care providers who have spent a long time with a patient or client feel like they are friends and object to this suggestion that they cannot be friends. This is more a semantic argument. In my mind a friend is someone who visits me and does not have to leave at the end of a "shift." Friends invite me to their homes, gossip about their work colleagues and bosses, and so much more. Paid staff and even volunteers are loyal to their service more than they can be to their patient or client.

The easiest way to determine whether you are a friend or a staff or volunteer is to decide if you would give up your position to remain loyal and more supportive to the person for whom you care. Since most of us cannot afford to do that for everyone we provide care to, it is best to concentrate on supporting and nurturing those relationships with families and friends that already exist or helping create new friendships for people isolated from their family and community.

6. Another aspect of this point is that some people, especially in smaller communities, may be friends first, or related to someone, for whom they are now providing professional care. This becomes more complicated in deciding which "hat" you are wearing when you are with the person. Nurses, for example, who are caring for a neighborhood friend (in the hospital or at home) must switch between being the friend to being the professional. They must deal with their own emotions while helping their friend professionally live as fully as possible until they die. Other care providers and family need to

recognize this difficulty and allow the person to fulfill both roles but at different times. Sometimes we feel most comfortable fulfilling our professional roles but we still need the support of others to go through the emotions of losing a dear friend during their final illness.

7. Help create memories using humor and creativity and a conspiracy of well-meaning people to help patients, their families and other caregivers. Memories are what we turn to in times of great difficulty and grief. We remember the good and the bad. A terminal illness gives us an opportunity to add new happy or profound memories for both the patients and their families and for other care providers. A few examples:

   (7.a) A young woman, 16 years old, was dying in a large university hospital. Her family were nearby but all her classmates were at least 5 hours away in her hometown. She knew and accepted that she was dying but she was clearly unhappy. The social worker helping her asked what was making her unhappy. The teenaged girl said she missed her friends. The social worker immediately understood. The social worker wanted to go the extra mile for her. So, after many phone calls to the girl's school principal and various other people, a school bus made the trip down to the city filled with the girl's friends. A special party was held in the hospital's auditorium. The girl knew her friends were coming so she made each and every one of them a special gift that she handed out at the party. Every person there from the patient, her family, all her friends, the bus driver, the principal, the social worker and other care providers all participated in something truly unique and wonderful. The memory of that event will last forever in the minds of everyone who attended and helped make it possible.

(7.b) Another example is a palliative care nurse who was caring for a young, recently married woman who had terminal uterine cancer. After many conversations together the nurse found out that the woman would dearly love to go to her favorite restaurant with her husband one more time. That was not possible given her condition however the nurse began to think of an alternative. She and another nurse rented tuxedoes and arranged for an ambulance to take the woman home for the evening. They had ordered food from the woman's favorite restaurant and served it (all dressed up as formal waiters!) in her own dining room. They did not chat with the young couple but served them as if they were in the restaurant. Then they quietly did the dishes and left the couple alone for a while. Then the ambulance came back later and returned the woman to the hospital where she died a few weeks later. Again, everyone who participated from the chef at the restaurant to the young couple and the nurses have a memory for a lifetime to share, relive and remember.

8. Volunteers have great opportunities to help. One man was visiting an elderly gentleman through a hospice program. The volunteer and the elder exchanged many stories during these visits to the point where the volunteer said, "Would you like me to help you record some of these stories as an legacy for your family?" The elder agreed and over a number of visits the volunteer used a tape recorder to record the stories which he then typed up on his home computer to create a "book," complete with scanned photos, for the elder to give to his family and friends on his 80th birthday. The legacy of this mutual gift will live on for generations through one volunteer's efforts.
9. Perfection is not possible. Perfect relationships do not exist. Conflicts will happen. However, when we compromise our care, for whatever reason, we must recognize the compromise so that it never becomes the preferred norm. For example, just because some people feel relief when they resolve a family dispute before they die does not mean that everyone who is dying should be coerced into trying to resolve

all family issues. [It's not possible, even if you tried!] Always stay focused on the individual's and family's needs rather than compare their situation to others you have already experienced. Start from scratch so that you don't impose your experiences onto them.

10. When people say their final goodbyes to the person who is dying, it can be very helpful to have someone else outside the room to give them a hug, offer a word of support, get them a cup of tea or whatever the person may find helpful and supportive. Saying goodbye is physically and emotionally painful. Anticipatory grief is equally painful. People who support someone who is dying also need support. Help each other. Comfort each other. This is part of the mutual gift of caring. Teach each other deep breathing techniques so that before you enter a patient's room, you slow your respiration and heart rate so that you become a calming presence rather than an anxious one.

IS IT BETTER TO GIVE THAN TO RECEIVE? NO!

The quote from the Bible about giving being better

than receiving (Acts 20:35) is based on sharing one's home, clothes and food with others in need. The hope is that one will share one's "things" with others so that no one goes without.

This concept of giving some of one's possessions to the poor is an admirable one. It has come to mean, however, that is better to help others than to ask for, or accept, help yourself. This lopsided view of care is one of the major reasons people refuse to accept help or refuse to ask for help from their own families and community services. They feel they are a burden rather than an equal partner in the mutual gift of care.

Ask yourself, would you rather offer and give support than ask for it or accept it yourself? How often in the past few years have you refused the help of others because you did not want to "burden" them or impose on them? How often do you refuse help because you think that accepting it would be a sign of weakness? If you answered 'yes' to any of these questions then you consciously or unconsciously view "caring" as an unequal relationship where only the care provider truly benefits.

When my father was in the ICU of a local

hospital on the brink of death (he survived and was able to come home to live until his death weeks later) I was standing in the waiting room talking with my fiancée. I do not know why I said it but I said, "You know, if ever this should happen to you, I will take care of you forever – I love you so much." Rather than leave well enough alone I then added, "But I am not sure I would want you to do the same for me."

I thought I was being thoughtful and considerate not expecting her to have to care for me should I get as ill as my father was at the time. She listened to what I had to say and then hit me. "How dare you think that you are a better person than I am!"

Of course, that is not what I was consciously trying to say at all. I was trying to say that I would care for her forever but that I would not ever want to be a burden to her if the roles were reversed. In hindsight, of course, I was saying exactly what she heard – "It is better to give than to receive care." I was saying that I would be a great husband but that I wouldn't expect her to be a great wife. How arrogant could I be? How arrogant are the rest of us who believe similar things?

I think it is dangerous to have such a belief. It forces people to refuse help and to die alone and lonely. It forces people to think they are burden when, in fact, they never viewed the people they cared for as burdens. It gives people an excuse not to allow people to feel as good about helping as they felt when they did it. It allows us to construct walls around us that we only choose to let people through on our terms.

The last gift we can give to others is the gift of allowing them to care for us. It really is that simple but certainly not always easy. I tell patients this all the time. At the end of our lives, we have the responsibility to allow people to care for us so they can learn the same wonderful knowledge and skills that we learned when we were providing the care. How can we expect our children and grandchildren to learn about what it means to care for someone if we only have allowed paid strangers to care for us?

One last example – a nurse came up to me after a presentation and told me about when her mother was dying. The nurse had two brothers and she was the only daughter. She took on the responsibility of caring for her mother at home while also having a family to raise herself working full time as a nurse. After a few months she became physically and emotionally exhausted. She could not do it anymore. So she called her brothers in and said, "I just can't take care of Mom alone anymore. You need to help."

"But we do help!" they answered. "We take care of the legal and financial stuff for Mom. We've prearranged her funeral. We've checked into how to sell the house after she dies. We are doing our piece."

The nurse answered, "That's all true but I can't physically provide all the home care that Mom needs and she can't get enough professional home care. I need more help with her personal care."

Now many men have very limited experiences with personal care of others. Some are getting used to helping with their babies but, on the whole, a lot of personal care of older children and older parents is still done by women. Where a husband is alive, however, most of them are providing the physical personal care to their wives so as not to "burden" the children.

The brothers understood their sister had

reached her end. With great fear that they would do it all wrong, they learned how to help their mother eat, help her get to the bathroom, and give her bed baths. They learned quickly that it was not hard compared to what they thought it would be like. In fact, the mother took the daughter aside one day and said, "I want Mike to give me my bed baths from now on. Is that okay?"

The nurse was partly hurt that something she was a 'professional' at was now being completely taken over by her brother. On the other hand she recognized how the bed baths were changing her brother's self-confidence and self-perception. The mother was giving her son the gift of care. She understood that her son would be a better husband, father and friend because of giving her the gift of a bed bath. Each learned, over some difficult hurdles, that this experience of caring for their mother was changing them as adults as well as changing them as siblings. The family became closer because of the care they provided their mother. There is no greater gift to a parent who is dying than watching her children become closer.

This closeness won't happen in every family, of

course. It is unrealistic to expect it. It is not unrealistic, however, to nurture it whenever you can and to nurture it within your own family always.

NO PEDESTALS PLEASE!

Have you ever been at a party and someone asks what you do? You mention that you care for people who are dying and they either immediately change the subject or they get that glazed look in their eyes of awe. They say something like, "Oh my goodness. I could never do that. You are so special. You must be like an angel to those people. You really are special."

Whether they actually say those words or it is their body language that says it, they are doing you and themselves a disservice.

When people want to raise you onto a pedestal because of how 'special' you are, what they are really doing is giving themselves an excuse never to have to try to provide personal care to someone they love. It implies that because you are so special, they do not have to make an effort to be supportive of someone going through grief. This belief that you must be trained and inherently "special" to be supportive makes them feel incompetent and not special enough to be the caregiver that they may well want to be.

In my case, had someone said to me, "Don't worry Harry. We'll take care of your mother for you," I probably would have been immensely grateful to them. I would not have learned what I was missing. As hard as providing care can be sometimes, there are also many wonderful gifts of care that go on. If you are not participating in that care, you cannot experience them. It is combining the best palliative medical care and personal support (through family and friends or through formal programs) that we all benefit.

Being on a pedestal can also be a very lonely experience for the person put up there. Do not allow people to think you are so special that you deserve to be up there on a pedestal. Remind them what it felt like when you first started – how incompetent you may have felt or frightened of doing the wrong things. Tell them of the good and the difficult. Tell them how life affirming the experiences have been while also being difficult. Encourage them to learn some basic home care techniques so they are ready when they need them. It is never too early to learn about physical, emotional, spiritual and information care in all health care situations.

Be a role model but one grounded in reality and within the hospice philosophy of care.

THE MOST DEADLY PHRASE

Each of us carries within our minds a phrase – the most deadly phrase in hospice palliative care. This phrase is:

I would rather be dead than have…

Each of us has a different ending to the phrases – perhaps many endings.

"I would rather be dead than ___________________.

have dementia

have cancer

have AIDS

have ALS

have heart disease

to lose a leg due to diabetes

to be poor, homeless, disabled, lonely, isolated, or

live in a long-term care facility.

How would you finish this phrase?

I would rather be dead than

____.

Why is this such a deadly phrase? How you fill in the blank above tells you which of your patients or clients are least likely to receive excellent care. If you would rather be dead than have cancer, how are you going to care for people who have cancer? Can you distance your own fears from the care you provide them?

If you would rather be dead than have dementia, what type of supports and outside help would you encourage for a patient who has dementia? How hard are you going to fight for supports when you think the patient, like you, would likely rather die than move to a long-term care facility or move in with a son or daughter? If the person had heart disease instead, perhaps you would advocate more strongly to get them the services and care they need. Since they have dementia, will that change how you advocate for them?

If you answer yes, that means you will likely find it hard to care for them as strongly as for someone who does not share your fear of this condition. Ensure to transfer this person to someone else's care. If you cannot transfer the patient who can likely provide better care how can you overcome your fear to provide life-affirming care when this person needs it most? How can you draw in their natural supports (e.g., family and friends) that will want to help the person live as fully as possible until they die?

Can you identify any fears you had when you were younger and how you overcame them? For example, I used to fear dementia a great deal. Then I saw some of the benefits of short-term memory loss in a man I used to visit. He had a horrible obstructed bowel that required difficult enemas on a regular basis. The nurse who performed these was always the same person. She always apologized for the discomfort she was causing him. What made the care easier for her was that he forgot who she was every time she visited. He also forgot the procedure he had within minutes of having it. He remembered much of his past and recognized his family but forgot, almost immediately, what he had eaten, what treatment he had, or who visited him earlier.

A daughter of a man who had Alzheimer's disease told me her story. Her grandmother had Alzheimer's disease so her father knew what to expect when he was diagnosed. His first comment to his family was, "This is going to be a lot harder for you guys than for me." He had already experienced what it was like when his mother became increasingly ill. He had led a very active and accomplished life rising to the top of his legal profession. His family was all grown up with grandchildren and he wanted to spare them some of the suffering he knew was awaiting them. In discussions with them, he described his own feelings as a son when he went through the experience with his mother. Then he discussed what would likely happen to him and how he felt his children and grandchildren could help. It was an open discussion. The discussion meant that the family was prepared for the imperfect last years with their father. There would be ups or downs. But they were somewhat prepared and they walked the final miles with him as best they could.

The father never said, "I would rather be dead than have Alzheimer's." He said, "Some of my care should be done by professionals so I am, at some point, going to move to the veterans' wing of the hospital. We can afford for me to stay at home but I want to help fellow veterans while I can. It may be sooner than you think I should go but I want to get to know the folks there and make a difference in their lives. That way they will also get used to me and what I need. I'll come home on weekends when I can until that becomes too difficult. Let's do this as best we can together."

Aside from how you would fill in the sentence "I would rather be dead then," there are other questions for you to consider:

1. What steps can you take to help overcome your own fears so that it will not impact the care you provide? This question will require some real effort and time to answer. Dealing with our fears is not a quick fix. It requires thoughtfulness, asking family and friends for help to look at coping strategies and, perhaps, professional help to identify and deal with your fears.
2. Who can you go to for help, guidance and mentorship?

3. How can you help others overcome similar fears?
4. Will you agree with decisions by other caregivers when they are more life affirming than your own decisions might be? If a patient has ovarian cancer and you believe they would be better off dead than alive, will you defer to the patient, family and those colleagues when they make difficult decisions that will likely lead to a longer life, regardless of the 'quality of life' as you see it?

"QUALITY OF LIFE"

The phrase "quality of life" is another deadly phrase. Originally it was used by researchers comparing whole populations of people. For example, they would compare people living in cities with those living in rural communities to compare their quality of life around issues of education, poverty, health care, nutrition, physical activities and such. It is possible to compare populations of people.

It is not, however, possible to evaluate what an individual person's quality of life is. You cannot measure, accurately, whether someone's life is worth living, nor can an individual measure that for themselves.

Someone who is grieving the death of a dear loved one would not rate their quality of life very high. Someone who has just lost a job or has discovered they have cancer, would rate their quality of life very high.

Similarly when we compare ourselves to other people, we often judge their lives as "not worth living." For example, if we were to evaluate someone's life who has a severe disability, is much older than us, is in prison or homeless, we would not rate their quality of life very high.

Yet those same people may well view their lives as very valuable and worth living.

When we impose a value of a good or a bad "quality of life" upon someone else we may encourage them to see their lives through our perspectives. If societally, we view people who have a disability as 'less valued' then they are at risk every time they go into hospital for care. If we view someone who is "too old" then we discourage them from treatments that might be very helpful.

I once had a journalist ask me if I would

treat an elderly man rushed into an Emergency Department with respiratory arrest?

I asked, "Is the man sick or dying?"

The journalist answered, "I don't know. It doesn't matter. He's old! Would you treat him?"

I replied that until I knew what was wrong with him, I would naturally treat him. At about the same time, an elderly woman (in her 90s I believe) was rushed to hospital in the UK with respiratory arrest. The doctors knew she was likely choking on a fish bone so obviously treated her without hesitation. She was also Queen Elizabeth's mother, the Queen Mum as she was affectionately referred to. She was a highly valued member of society and so was treated without reservation. I wonder what the journalist would have done in similar circumstances? I bet she would have treated the Queen Mum too, even though she "was old!"

That is why "quality of life" is such a deadly phrase. We use it to compare people to ourselves and justify actions that are not justifiable. We cannot measure a person's worth at any specific point in their life. The day after a difficult surgery with the patient experiencing complications is not a good day to judge their 'quality of life' any more than judging them on their wedding day would be an accurate description of their lives.

We must avoid this phrase and the thinking behind it at all costs.

There are now evaluation scales used for costing analysis of a person's quality of life. One is called the *Quality-Adjusted Life Years (QALY)* which equals the number of expected years to live and presumed satisfactory quality of life which leads to the cost-per-QALY point index!

A group of 247 neonatologists in the U.S. were surveyed with the majority saying that babies of women with HIV should be allowed to die because the babies would have a poor quality of life, even if the babies were not infected. (*Syracuse Herald Journal*, June 12, 1991) That conclusion would not, I hope, be the same today, but it was then. Today it would be more likely for babies born with various types of disabilities who would be "better off dead" because their future quality of life would be so poor.

In the Netherlands, a TV documentary interviewed doctors at a hospital where many pre-mature babies were treated. The head physician said that, although they didn't tell the parents, they let boys born with deformed penises die because their future quality of life would be so poor. They told the parents that their baby died because of complications.

IDENTIFYING YOUR LIMITS

There is an exercise I do with participants in my workshops. I ask them to close their eyes and imagine one or more of their patients or clients. I play some music in the background so that they can quietly answer the following questions to put their care into perspective.

There are limits to what we can do for people. There are also limits to what patients and their families can do for us. When we identify them, we may feel less anxious that we are not doing enough and we can, perhaps, reduce our expectations of those we care for. Here are the questions:

1. What is it that I can do to help patients and families?
2. What is it that I cannot do, no matter how

much I wish I could?

3. What is it that patients and families can do to help me?
4. What is it that they cannot do, no matter how much they wish they could?

Let us look at each one more carefully.

1. What is it that I can do to help patients and families?

Here you can identify both your knowledge and skills that can help a patient and their families but also a list of the personal attributes you bring to someone – your beliefs, your assumptions and how you can help them nurture the relationships important in their lives. You are an individual with individual tastes and talents. Identify those that can be helpful to a specific patient and their family.

2. What is it that I cannot do, no matter how much I wish I could?

There are some things you cannot do either because they are beyond your experience or skills or because they go beyond your own personality or beyond the circumstances. For example, you cannot pretend to belong to a person's faith when you have a different one. You will need to bring in others from the person's own faith community to help meet some of their specific spiritual needs. That does not prevent you from sharing some aspects in common between all faiths but it does limit you in following some of the traditional rights and rituals of the patient's faith. Another example may be that you would like to help the family resolve decades-old conflicts but you have neither the skill nor time to do it well. It may be something you would like to do, but you cannot in these circumstances.

3. What is it that patients and families can do to help me?

Part of the philosophy of care described in this book is that care, to be truly effective, must have mutual elements to it. That means, it is not better to give than to receive, therefore, patients and their families must be allowed to give back to you in some ways. What ways might that be so that they can help you with your work? Several examples: if you are coming to provide personal care, any family members present could have all the necessary towels, soaps, etc. ready for you and they can offer to help with the personal care so they can learn from you. If you are a volunteer coming over to help the person respond to letters they have received, the person or family could have the letters, cards, stamps, pens and such laid out for you or they might make you a cup of tea while you work with the patient. This sense of mutual care can be very practical or it can also be that they give you a warm smile when you visit or a hug of thanks or a homemade cookie. It is about sharing in the care in whatever ways are possible.

4. What is it that they cannot do, no matter how much they wish they could?

One of the things that patients cannot do for you, even if they really wanted to, is to get well. This may seem an odd thing to say to a professional or volunteer palliative care provider. But sometimes, that is exactly what we wish the patients would do – get well. How can you identify when this is happening to you? Perhaps you want to try to feed a patient who is no longer hungry. You might see desire for the patient to get well in your colleagues (professional or volunteer). For example, you may see someone try to get a life-long smoker to quit (as they did with my father who had emphysema) in the last weeks of their life. In fact, this hurts the patient as smoking actually increased their intact of oxygen (through the deep breathing in that smokers do). A family member might encourage a patient to try the latest alternative medicine regime in hopes that it might work. All of these things are ways to tell the patient that we want them to try harder to get well and all of them, likely, will be unsuccessful and even unkind.

There are other things that patients and families cannot do for us even though they may wish to. For example, they cannot fix the health care system that expects too much from too few staff and volunteers. They cannot find enough money to safeguard your program. They cannot find the energy in their last weeks, likely, to always smile and "be happy" when you come to visit. Your expectations of them have to be realistic to the circumstances, no matter how much they would actually like to meet your spoken and unspoken expectations.

So put on some quiet music, put your feet up and enjoy a warm cup of tea or a cool glass of your favorite drink and think about the answers to these four questions for yourself. It is important that you know what your limits are and the limits of those you care for so that you use your knowledge, skills and energies to their best.

CHAPTER 3

Helpful Assumptions to Hold and Role Model

Some of you reading this book will have administrative or political influence in how your program and services are provided. Others of you are direct bedside professionals, family members, and volunteer care providers.

Each of you will have influence over the types of services that the actual patient and their families receive. Because of your influence, it is important that you have certain helpful assumptions in designing and providing your care. You may not be able to control all aspects of the care delivered to your patients and their families, but you can greatly impact on their lives through your own assumptions and actions. Some of these assumptions are so obvious you may feel like skipping over them. Remember, that you are a guardian of the modern hospice movement and that what is obvious to you is not obvious to your patients, their families, members of the community and those with political control over your program. The more you can speak about these assumptions, the more likely others with begin to use them in making life and death decisions over your patients.

1. Death is a natural process--a part of living.
2. Each life is valued and should be preserved and supported to its natural end.
3. People can have valued roles until they die (i.e., maintain or enhance typical roles such as parent, spouse, child or friend).
4. Whenever possible, concentrate on enhancing natural supports (family, friends, neighbors) versus program supports.
5. Servers should be loyal to the person and family who is ill rather than to their service.
6. The person receiving service, the server and society all benefit from the relationship.
7. The spiritual foundation of hospice care is fundamental to its success as it reminds us of its roots, its basic philosophy and our need to

put patients and families above systemic and bureaucratic needs.

Let us look at each of these:

1. Death is a natural process – a part of living. The hospice movement began in part because many people were dying in Intensive Care Units where every thing was done to save a person's life even if they were obviously dying.

People were force fed, given ineffective and painful test and treatments, and isolated from their loved ones all in the futile attempt to save their lives. Death or dying was not discussed as this was too time consuming and physicians and nurses were often very uncomfortable with the topic themselves. After all, it was never part of their training. To see death as a natural process was, in fact, seen as "giving up" and, therefore, not acceptable. More and more people now acknowledge this basic assumption of dying but it is certainly not a universal assumption.

2. Each life is valued and should be preserved and supported to its natural end.

We know that some people 'naturally' receive better care than others. It is mostly a subconscious process but in many cases it is also very overt. People with mental illnesses, for example, are less likely to receive support to live to their natural end. Elderly people are often assumed to be wanting to die so will not be offered certain treatments and care that will prolong their lives in the same way as someone with a similar condition who is younger.

As I wrote previously, a reporter once asked me what I would do if an elderly person came into the Emergency Unit of the hospital and I was the physician attending to them. Would I provide life-supporting treatment to them? I asked the reporter if the elderly person was ill? The reporter replied, "I don't know. They are just old. Would you treat them?" My answer was that until I knew what was wrong with them that I would, of course, treat the person. The reporter could not understand my answer. Why would you treat an old person? The answer to that is this assumption that each life is valued and should be preserved and supported to its natural end – not prolonged painfully or cruelly; neither shortened based on our often misguided perceptions of what the person wants or needs.

3. ***People can have valued roles until they die (i.e., maintain or enhance typical roles) to ensure they get better treatment.***

Earlier in the Introduction to this book you read about Mr. G and his granddaughter who saw the whole man rather than the ugly tumor covering the lower part of his face. This granddaughter reminded everyone that this patient was also a husband, a father, a grandfather and friend to many others. These were some of his valued roles that he, and those caring for him, had forgotten. This assumption of maintaining and enhancing one's typical and valued roles is about seeing beyond their physical, emotional and spiritual condition and helping them to live fully until they die. Role modeling this approach is one of your most powerful gifts of care.

When my father was diagnosed with cancer he was forced to quit his work. He was still able to work but the label of cancer frightened his young employer who told my father he needed to retire "for his own good." This changed my father's role from property manager to cancer patient. It changed his daily routine from one of a valued worker to one of a patient waiting to die. Like so many other people in similar situations, his life was probably shortened when his perceived value was diminished. Although he was still a father and grandfather, he saw himself as less valuable. Medically, he was no longer the patient who arrived in a business suit with years of work life ahead of him but an emotionally diminished man awaiting his death.

As a professional or volunteer caregiver, as well as family members and friends, your life affirming perspective will help people like my father. You can help them deal with the real debilitating grief of job loss while helping them recognize the practical ways in which their lives still matter as parent, grandparent, sibling, friend, neighbor and fellow patient. There is much that patients have to offer but they often need someone else to tell them what that is.

When they recognize these 'gifts' they have yet to offer, they are more likely to arrive for medical appointments and treatments with hope that in turn often leads to better care.

4. *Whenever possible, concentrate on enhancing natural supports (family, friends, neighbors) versus program supports.*

Many people have at least a few people around them who care but who are afraid of doing or saying the wrong thing. How you treat and speak with the patient in front of their loved ones is one way to enhance the natural supports available to the patient. When a spouse or adult child sees you give a bed bath, they listen to the words you use and the compassionate body language you project. They learn from you. When they see that when you sit beside the patient rather than remain standing and looking down on the patient, they will copy you. When a patient needs a stronger advocate because of their circumstances, you can provide their loved ones with specific ideas, language and questions to ask of the right people so that the patient receives the care they deserve.

For example, when you ask specific questions about pain and symptom control, families will learn the type of questions to ask. More importantly, they will learn that such questions are okay to ask. When you suggest that a patient and their family request a second opinion, it shows that such request are normal and acceptable. When you suggest that a family member always attend all medical appointments and that they take notes, you are giving them permission to ask questions and record answers so that you can help the patient understand the information during and after the appointment.

5. ***Servers should be loyal to the person who is ill and their family rather than to their service.***

If a service would actually allow their staff and volunteers to be truly loyal to their patient first, then you could advocate as strongly as you would like. However, that is likely not the case for many reasons. However, if you assume that your loyalty is first with the patient, even if in reality it cannot be because you need the job, then you will see areas where you can advocate more strongly while also nurturing loved ones to fulfill an even stronger advocacy role when you cannot. This is the main reason to strengthen a person's natural supports

– because they can be loyal to the person first.

6. The person receiving service, the server and society all benefit from the relationship.

Many people believe in the adage "it is better to give then to receive." Because of this assumption, providing care is often seen as a 'charitable' act rather than as a mutual gift of care. As a charitable act, the program and services you provide can be easily cut when 'higher' priorities require the resources. When people see that the patient, server and society all benefit from the hospice care relationship, society and governments are less likely to cut funding, diminish the importance of your care and, perhaps, even recognize that all dying patients are only slightly farther ahead in the line-up to death than they are.

7. The spiritual foundations of hospice care are fundamental to its success. They remind us of its roots, its basic philosophy and our need to put patients and families above systemic and bureaucratic needs.

Spirituality has to do with who we are as people. Religion has to do with how we practice our spirituality, if at all, through various religious beliefs, practices and rituals. We are all spiritual people in the sense that we all have a need to know our lives have value and meaning. We are all children of God, however we describe God, and we are connected to each other, and to all nature, as members of a living community.

The only thing that separates us spiritually is our belief that separateness is possible. Our spirituality is often best expressed in times of great joy or distress. It is felt during moments of genuine bliss when we watch our baby sleep, see a sunset from our favorite mountain, or listen to the calm of a summer breeze.

All ancient spiritual beliefs have similar principles of compassionate care for those who are dying. Whatever your spiritual belief and traditions, use them to remind yourself of the unique opportunities that hospice palliative care provides you to make a real difference in someone's life everyday. Modern health care has divided physical care from emotional and spiritual care. Traditionally physicians and nurses were often seen praying with their patients, fluffing their pillows with a kind heart, helping them on with their clothes after an examination and so much more. They had the common bond of being children of God, however they defined God. In modern times, this unique human bond has been separated so there is a clear "us" and a clear "them." Even health care providers themselves, when they are patients, remark on how different they feel and how isolating and fearful those differences can be. It is only when they are treated as people first rather than patients that they feel comfortable lying on the patient bed.

QUESTIONS TO ASK YOURSELF

To evaluate what you do and the impact it has on your patients, their families, your colleagues and your own family, take a few minutes to answer these questions.

1. Who is benefiting most from the palliative care services provided? Is it really the patient and their family or are the staff, volunteers, government and other funding agencies benefiting most?

How can you tell? Are staff and volunteers spending more time with each other than with patients and families? Are government and other funding agencies providing the funding because they truly care for the patients' needs or are they providing only sufficient funding so they can 'prove' that they are doing something to the voting public? Are the funders so active in the running of the program and services that the organization can no longer provide the care that they used to provide so well.

2. What are the values your program uses in developing, applying and evaluating your services? Are they coherent? By coherent I mean, are these values known, disseminated, internalized, and safeguarded with checks and balances to discourage abuse of the patient and their family? Do the values lead directly to practical approaches to care that affirm the importance of the patient's life until they die a natural death? When people are uncertain of what to do, do they revert back to these values to decide what to do next? For example, is there a strong stance against institutionalizing patients except as a last resort? Are the patients, family and friends recognized and helped to provide mutual

care? Are emotional and spiritual supports seen as more important than high tech alternatives?

3. Is professionalization of hospice palliative care overtaking your work and destroying the essence of knowing the people you serve, knowing your colleagues and knowing the community? In other words, are the staff and volunteers professionalized and specialized and segregated to the point that people in the community cannot possibly imagine themselves capable of helping their loved ones through their last illness?

4. How are patient needs assessed and taken into account to ensure their physical, emotional, spiritual and information needs are met? Are the actual needs of the patient taken into account rather than using a standard assessment process that misses many of these points?

For example, my great aunt was a Catholic nun. When she was dying she refused all pain medication saying, "I came into this world without drugs and I will leave without them too. I will be comforted by my faith and by God." A standard assessment of her may well have identified her need for spiritual control over her death or it could have labelled her with all sorts of terms that would have prevented her from living out her life as she had thoughtfully decided. Her assessment form may have had words like non-compliant, in denial, requires psychiatric assessment, and more. The convent where she lived supported her decisions and cared for her through what many would have called a difficult, painful death. She died, however, as she wished and was supported fully by her religious community. Does your service provide as much personal control to your patients?

Once you have answered these questions for yourself, consider sharing your conclusions with your colleagues to see what they think. People can never think or belief in exactly the same thing or act in exactly the same ways but they can be encouraged to see how their beliefs can help, or harm, the people for whom they care. You can be that catalyst.

THE MOST FUNDAMENTAL HOSPICE CARE QUESTION TO ANSWER

When I teach hospice palliative care courses at colleges and universities I hand out the final exam question on the first day of classes. I tell the students that at the end of the course, they will be asked to write an essay answering this single question:

Why would someone near the end of life
want you in the same room with them?

They are told to answer this question with complete honesty and within the context of their personal and professional/volunteer life.

To help you answer this fundamental question, use the chart on the following page to identify your beliefs and assumptions. Our beliefs and assumptions impact our conscious and unconscious behaviors. Each strength you have, such as a "giving spirit," can turn into something harmful. If you give so much of yourself that you do not allow others to give back, you have turned a strength into something harmful.

Another example of how any of your strengths can turn out to be harmful is a woman that I met at a workshop for volunteer chaplaincy workers at a hospital. I had presented to a group that was half Christian and half Muslim. During a break this Christian woman came up to me and said, "They very nice aren't they?" I answered, "Who?" "Those Muslim people over there. They're really nice aren't they? But you know what, they will never get to heaven."

Her comment was not distressing because of her belief of who would and would not get to heaven. Many people have beliefs that are different than my own. What was distressing was that she was a chaplaincy volunteer in a hospital that had a very diverse population of patients within it. I spoke with her and her Director of Chaplaincy to ensure that this volunteer would only ever be assigned a patient with her specific faith. That didn't mean assigned only to Christian patients. It meant that she would only be assigned Christian patients of her specific denomination. A person's faith cannot be questioned on the basis of right and wrong. It can however inform you as to whether the person would be comfortable with only patients of their specific faith or with people of many different faiths. Her faith was a great strength and comfort to her. Her faith would also harm patients who did not share in her faith and who might be spoken to about how they could convert, before they died, so they too could get to heaven.

Once we know our beliefs and assumptions we are better able to answer "Why would someone near the end of life want you in the same room with them?"

As a background to the question, imagine yourself lying in your bed at home looking up at the ceiling. Surrounding your bed are the people you love most in life. Imagine their faces looking down at you. They are watching you breathe and, actually, they are waiting for when you are no longer breathing. This is your deathbed. Given that is the scenario for most of the people you care for, why would they, or should they, be introduced to you at such a time in their lives? Why would they want you in that room with them? Of course, many of you will know the patients before they get to this stage, but the question remains – why would they want you present over someone else? Why should they have to say goodbye to one more person in their lives when it is hard enough to say goodbye to the people who are already there?

IMPACT OF YOUR BELIEFS/ASSUMPTIONS

Look at each heading in the chart below and evaluate how any of your assumptions and beliefs can both help and, hinder other people – those you care for as well as those you work with.

QUESTION	ANSWER	MAY HELP or HARM Others
What assumptions about life and death do you strongly adhere to? e.g. freedom of choice, sanctity of life, elders are to be respected and listened to vs. elders must be protected.		
What elements of care are you most comfortable in providing: physical, emotional, spiritual, advocacy?		

QUESTION	ANSWER	MAY HELP or HARM Others
Where do you feel most comfortable in practicing your profession: person's home, residential setting, hospital, LTC facility?		
Do you see your relationship with your clients as care giving or mutual caring?		
What do you fear most about providing service to clients? How do you deal with your fears?		
What gives you comfort when you are under a lot of stress?		

QUESTION	ANSWER	MAY HELP or HARM Others
What can you do for others? What can you not do for them? What can they do for you? What can they not do for you?		
Have you ever "walked in the shoes" of a client to understand their experiences?		

When you look at the assumptions presented early on in this chapter along with your answers in the chart above, how will you answer: **Why would someone near the end of life want you in the same room with them?**

CHAPTER 4

Understanding Your Family Member/Patients/Clients

COMMON EXPERIENCES

Most of your patients and their families have similar experiences throughout the course of a final illness. They will likely have experienced a 'roller coaster' of their highest highs and lowest lows that are life defining. Such experiences encourage them, their families and, perhaps, their care providers to re-define their life priorities with more emphasis on putting their energies into nurturing the relationships they value most.

Most of them will say that looking back on their lives, they have discovered that it was these relationships they have had that were most important to them and have provided the greatest comfort in their last months. It was not the "things" they have accumulated or the accomplishments they have achieved but the people they have loved that has made the greatest difference. As care providers many family members feel that they learned to be a better child, spouse, parent, friend, and neighbor.

On the down side of this roller coaster are often experiences such as a lack of diagnosis for many weeks if not months, tests and tests and more tests (often painful or at least uncomfortable), uncertainty about the future, successful and failed treatments (medical and alternative), painful and uncomfortable symptoms and the final news that they have a terminal illness. For the lucky few they may have also been referred early on for adequate pain and symptom control through a program offering the hospice palliative philosophy of care.

The patients, their families and their professional and volunteer care providers will all experience a range of human emotions including laughter, tears, silence, rage, joy, fear, love, awe, horror and touch.

INDIVIDUAL DIFFERENCES

Just as there are common experiences for most of your patients and their families there are also individual differences. A person's age, birth order, culture, gender, historical and family backgrounds, religion, their previous experiences of the death of loved ones, their social roles (a valued or devalued member of their community), the degree of unfinished business in their lives, other recent losses, their personal beliefs and personal wants and regrets all impact their experience.

To truly help them as individuals requires two levels of understanding. In the short term, concentration on their basic, self-expressed needs is most important. There is little good in trying to help them deal with cultural isolation if there are experiencing horrible pain. Their top priorities must be met first and this usually includes relief of unbearable pain and nurturing existing relationships so the person is not alone or feeling as if they are a burden.

After the immediate needs are met, and if you have a longer time with patients (months as opposed to days or a few weeks) then you may be able to help them with other needs. You may be able to bring together their family to work out long-standing difficulties. You may be able to draw in their spiritual community to help them with their spiritual needs. You may be able to help them arrange some of their legal, financial and funeral preparations affairs.

At all times, you can model the hospice palliative care philosophy of care so that others can learn by your example.

PEOPLE'S FEARS

In helping someone with their immediate needs, it is important to start by **understanding their fears**. They may be so afraid of inadequate pain control, yet convinced by family history that it is inevitable and they just have to suffer through, that they will not know to ask for help with their pain. People of some cultures in particular have this stoic attitude as part of their family history. To help them meet their most basic needs, therefore, it is important to understand their individual fears.

People do not experience all the following fears but they may experience one or more of them at different times during their illness. Understanding these fears makes it easier to provide them that extra minute or two of compassionate care that so many people crave.

People may fear having unbearable pain

Most people have seen their loved ones experience terrible pain before they died. They expect the same to happen to them. If you have ever seen something curl up in a fetal position, rock back and forth and pray to die because the pain is so great, you will understand why this fear of pain looms large in people's minds. Let them know that hospice palliative care's first credo is the relief of unbearable pain and symptoms and ensure their pain and symptoms are well controlled as soon as possible. Once you have shown them what is possible, they are more likely to believe you about others aspects of care that you can help them with. If you are a volunteer, advocate as strongly as possible that the proper medical care providers get involved so that the person's immediate suffering is relieved. No one needs suffer unbearable pain and symptoms. No one.

People may fear being a "burden"

Often the second most common fear of patients is their sense of being a burden to their loved ones and others. They would rather suffer in isolation in their own homes than let their families know they need help and support. They would rather lay in a hospital bed in extreme pain than "bother the nice nurses." They would rather go without food in the fridge than ask a neighbor to pick up a few groceries. They would rather soil their pants than ask a family member's help in going to the bathroom. And, in fact, many would rather die than lose their 'dignity' by requiring toileting help at all.

These people need reassurance that dignity is not defined by how much help one needs to go to the bathroom. They may need someone to talk to their families about these fears. They need reassurance that providing care and support may be difficult sometimes for family and friends but that they would much rather provide that care than see the person go without. They need to understand that juggling time management priorities for families is not the same thing as wishing the patient was dead. They need to be reminded that caring for one's family and friends is part of daily life; not an exception to living. They also need to be reminded that they received wonderful benefits from helping others in need during their life times so why would they think to take the opportunity away from those they love most.

People may fear how they look throughout their illness (their body image)

As a society we are very critical when it comes to how people look. For example, we often tell young girls and women that they need all sorts of make up, special hairdos, particular clothes to look beautiful. When we are told that someone is ill in hospital or at home we immediately tell them it doesn't matter if they hair hasn't been washed in a week, or that they are not wearing their usual make up, or that their nails have not been cared for. We say, "You look beautiful just the way you are."

Sick people do not become stupid because of their illness. They know they look "sick" and they know instinctively that they would "feel" better if they looked better. So helping them with their personal hygiene, washing and setting their hair, applying makeup that is not sensitive to their medical treatment (e.g., some makeup reacts negatively with some medications), doing their nails (hands and feet), and letting them wear clothes in which they feel most comfortable are all wonderful gifts of care.

People may fear the progress of their illness

Many people fear how their illness will progress. Will it take too long (and therefore be a greater burden to their family)? Will it be painful? Will they end up looking like concentration camp victims?

This last fear of becoming severely emaciated is a modern fear. Before World War II and those horrible photos of concentration camp victims, people expected that as their bodies slowed down they would eat less and naturally lose weight. Perhaps they did not "look" great, but there was no stigma attached to this natural process of their bodies slowing down. After the war, the images of how much the prisoners suffered in these camps forever became tied to the look of dying people. The stigma is very strong and people fear their emaciated look will frighten themselves but more importantly their families.

This is where your reassurance and planning come in. Concentration camp survivors and victims did not live in their own homes. They were not surrounded by loving families. They could not wear comfortable clothes and receive food and drink upon request. They had no recreational activities or family events to look forward to. They were completely isolated from anything that might be perceived as compassionate care.

You are there to remind the patients that their grandparents and great grandparents experienced the same natural slowing down of their bodies as they will likely experience. You are there to help them plan to have different kinds of clothes to cover how they look. You are there to help families understand the natural process that is going on and how they should try to avoid comparing their loved one who is ill with the historical photos they have seen. For those who are there daily, this will not be very hard to do as they will see the changes happening very slowly. For those who may not see the person for several weeks or months the difference in how the person looks will be more dramatic. Help prepare them for how the person has changed and, perhaps, tell them the person who is ill is not different inside other than, perhaps, a bit wiser about the importance of relationships versus the importance of how one looks. Remember the story of Mr.

G earlier in this book to remind yourself of how a six-year old granddaughter reminded everyone of the importance of her grandfather in her life.

People may fear losing control and being increasingly dependent on others

This fear partly relates to be a burden to one's family. However, some people fear losing control and being dependent even if they families and care providers have no sense of burden at all. The person who is ill may have been used to being in control most of their lives and find losing that control immensely painful and frightening.

Above all else they need opportunities to feel in control during uncontrollable times. For example, my grandfather, at the age of 92, when he was dying decided one day that he no longer wanted to be presented with food. He only wanted water with some sugar in it (a sweet tooth to the end!). He had eaten very little over the previous weeks and really did not feel the need to eat anymore. He was dying and knew it and did not want the taste or smell of foods in his bedroom anymore. He added, "Even if I ask for food, don't give it to me."

Those of us caring for him (two of his daughters and myself) wondered if this was a good idea at first. We believed, as so many do, that eating will give you health and would help my grandfather live longer. After a short discussion we recognized that he really was near his end and to try to force or coerce him to eat was just wrong. So we agreed with his request.

The next day when I was in the room with him he said, "I'd like a ham sandwich, please." When I told my aunts they wondered if he was having short-term memory loss and that he forgotten about his request the previous day. We brought him the sandwich, however, and he took one bite and asked us to take it away. He said with a twinkle in his eyes, "I just wanted to see if you would give it to me."

He was a conservative businessman who had been in control of his business and family for all of his adult life. He was used to being in control and his illness had robbed him of much of that control. This one act helped him regain some personal sense of control and the beam on his face reflected the inner joy he had in having some of his control back.

Anytime you can give a patient or their families

a sense of control in a period where so much control is taken away, you are providing the gift of care. Even the flow of information can be based on this simple principle. If you have information that may be difficult or discomforting for the person, offer them control over when they will hear the information.

For example, you might say, "You have to decide soon about whether or not you are going to have that treatment the doctor spoke to you about yesterday. Would you like to discuss your decision now, later this afternoon or perhaps tomorrow morning?" There are few decisions that cannot wait 24 hours and by giving the patient 3 choices from which to choose they have a sense of control during difficult times. Many just want a bit of time to prepare for difficult news or decisions while others want to know immediately and decide immediately. That sense of control gives them not only some emotional support but also, perhaps, more self-confidence to withstand whatever will happen next.

People may fear dealing with the unknown

How often have you heard someone say after finding out a diagnosis that they are "relieved" to finally know what they are dealing with? My mother went through months of tests and uncertainty before she found out she had terminal cancer.

During those months of uncertainty, however, she was often made to feel as if her condition was "all in your head." They did the tests more to "soothe" her concerns than they did because they believed something was wrong. Dealing with the unknown is very debilitating physically, emotionally and even spiritually.

During times of uncertainty, families and care providers can help the person reclaim control over other aspects of their care and their lives. You cannot erase the uncertainty but you can ensure that they are not alone with uncertainty for long periods or that their concerns are unwarranted. Because no one knows what they are dealing with, the uncertainty affects everyone.

This is the time when nurturing natural and loving relationships can be most important. You may have to wait until two or four or six months before you know what is wrong or what is likely to happen, but those months can be extraordinarily special if you use them to create memories of love, joy, laughter, closeness, hugs and adventure.

These are also times when a person may choose to research their condition themselves or ask you to help them find out what might be happening. The Internet has opened up a whole new world of information that used to be limited to only a few professionals. When doing the research or helping someone do it, ensure you are using websites that are known for excellent information. Determine which sites have traditional information and which may be suggesting alternative and complementary treatments. Check the resources at the end of this book for some examples. Websites change regularly so use your browser to search for new reliable ones as well.

People may fear losing loved ones

It is not just families that begin to grieve the loss of their loved one before they die. The patient also begins to grieve the loss of their future without the people they love. Some people may be of an age or experience where death is not as traumatic as for others. For many, however, saying goodbye to loved ones stretched over weeks and months takes its physical and emotional toll. Recognition of what professionals call "anticipatory grief" is a beginning to help minimize some of the effects. As long as a person is living they can be encouraged to fulfil their role as spouse, parent, sibling, grandparent and friend. Family members can be encouraged to resolve outstanding issues understanding that not all will become resolved. Each person involved is given the gift of time to ensure that they say what they have wanted to say, that they hold the person for as long as they can, that they create new memories of love and that they have few regrets upon the person's death.

For the patient, they are given this gift of time to do much of the same but also to get their affairs in order, to give gifts to each and every person they love whether the gift be something they want to give them (e.g., special books, artwork, jewelry) or the gift of stories either written out or given verbally.

This is a time when the patient can talk about

their hopes and dreams for their loved ones. Although families often don't want to talk about the future without their loved one in it, the patient does. They have things to say, advice to offer and dreams to share. These are often very emotional conversations but what a gift they are.

People may fear causing loved ones fear and suffering

In a similar vein as worrying about being a burden, feeling like you will cause your loved ones fear and suffering is often very difficult for patients. Not only do they not want to be a burden, they do not want their final illness to cause discomfort, fear or suffering. To watch a child cope with a parent's terminal illness is one example. To imagine the concern a husband of 50 years has when he is dying and how his wife will cope is another. The patient almost believes that it would all be so much easier for everyone if they just died quickly.

However, it is not easier – it is different. People who die suddenly leave behind families and friends who never got a chance to say goodbye. They never got a chance to resolve any conflicts.

They are often left with various degrees of guilt for things unsaid or undone. They may not have to face the days, weeks or even months of day-to-day care, but they also get little support after a week or two from their family, friends and colleagues to "get over" the death. When a person lives a longer time through their last illness, their families and friends are likely to receive more support for their emotional roller coaster.

There is no "better" way to die. Each has its own consequences. For the patient, however, dying suddenly may feel like it is easier and, for them, it might be as they do not have to watch their loved ones cope with the illness. They do not have to try and help them prepare for a life without them.

On the other hand, if the patient dies quickly they also lose out on the opportunity to say the things they have always wanted to say; to do the things they may have put off for too long and to live in the comfort of more hugs, moments of genuine love and experience the transition from life to death to after death in all its possibilities.

Your role becomes helping them identify what is possible rather than on concentrating on the negative aspects of their circumstances. Help them be hopeful for what they can accomplish today rather than concentrate on what they can no longer do. Help them identify how they can continue to make a difference in the lives of their loved ones even when they may feel that their loved ones would rather have them die more quickly.

People may fear isolation and abandonment

Many people fear being left alone and abandoned at the end of their lives. This is especially true of surviving spouses and single people without a lot of family close by. Reassurance that they are not alone is not enough. They have seen, especially many women, all too often where their friends have been abandoned by their loved ones either intentionally (dysfunctional relationships) or unintentionally (family and friends live far away). The latter is most common when a couple moves from where they have lived for decades to "retire" to a different community far from those who love them most.

In my books *Caring for Loved Ones at Home* (a basic home nursing guide for family and friends) and *Family Hospice Care* (a pre-planning and hospice palliative care guide) there is a chapter on how to set up support circles to ensure that no one is left alone at the end of their lives. The chapters provide specific planning steps to take to provide people with a circle of people who will be there around the clock if necessary while minimizing the intrusiveness of such constant care. People do not have to be alone but it takes some thoughtful planning and the hospice palliative care philosophy to make it work best for everyone involved.

People may fear having had a meaningless life

When we are younger, we presume to know more than we do and we believe we have all the answers. We have a "clean slate" before us to plan our lives any way we think best. We can change careers (the average is now between 3-5 careers for each of us), change our families and friends, change our location to almost anywhere in the world and change our personalities.

At the other end of life, we may feel "stuck" with our history and all the decisions we have made. We may feel "stuck" with the family and friends that we have now (no time to make new ones) and we may feel "stuck" by where we live. Mostly, we may feel dissatisfied with how "it" (our life) has unfolded. We probably thought we had more time to do things differently. We may have regrets and we may feel guilt over past actions.

Almost all of us will have some of the above. What can you do as a supportive care provider?

There are two areas of our lives we have control over: how we focus on our past and what we do with the remainder of our present and future. You can help the patient review their past looking at both the good and the bad. Helping them record some of their life stories as a family heirloom is one way to help. (see: *Recording Your Life and Family Stories*). You may help them write to, or speak with, their loved ones to recognize the good and the bad of their relationships and the patient's hopes and dreams for their loved ones' futures. You can help them use their remaining days to their utmost so that each day offers opportunities for them to create lasting memories of love, joy, adventure and meaning.

You can also tell the person how they have changed your life. Regardless of how someone has lived, it is how they live in their last months that offers them a unique opportunity to teach their life's wisdom as they have learned it. Each person I have cared for offered me wisdom in this way.

My mother (53 years old when she died) taught me that finding a kindred spirit with whom to share my life with was my most important task. She had found hers and that helped her through the death of their first born child, moving to a new country without speaking the language or having a job waiting for them, raising children in the difficult years of the 60s and 70s when so much of society was changing at breakneck speed and more.

My grandfather (92 years old when he died) taught me that one is never too old to change. At the age of 78 he went to each of his 9 surviving children and apologized for any mistakes he made in raising them. He knew he had been too strict and that work too often took precedence over his family. He asked for their forgiveness and hoped that they would not make the same mistakes with their children.

My father (59 when he died) sat me down one day and told me with tears in his eyes "No one is better than you son. You must believe enough in yourself to understand that. But, at the same time, you must always know that you are not better than anyone else either. We are all equal." He taught me that we each have gifts to share and that, thankfully, we do not all have the same gifts. It is finding out how we complement each other that we end up making the greatest difference in the lives of others and ourselves.

These are incredible lessons to learn. All of them, and the many which followed, taught me to concentrate my life on nurturing relationships because, at the end of life, they are all that will sustain and comfort you. They also taught that it is never too late to try and nurture past relationships and even have a few new ones with care providers who genuinely care for you. Your nurturing may not always be accepted at the moment, but the effort will have a lasting impact on everyone you know and love.

Each of these fears is real for the people who have them. It is not enough to brush them aside because you have seen them too often before. Each must be addressed to the person's satisfaction as much as possible. These fears are often based on experiences with the deaths of loved ones who were isolated, or perceived as burdensome or who felt a real lose of control over their life and death.

Once fears are out in the open, their power diminishes and alternative resources can help to overcome the fears. As long as they are private, their effects will be felt. Therefore, from these fears we can identify some basic **human needs** that shared by all of us.

PEOPLE'S NEEDS

People's needs are individual yet there are trends of needs that most people have including the need to feel safe and loved. The following list provides an extensive sample of the types of needs that people have. Helping people meet their needs deals directly with helping them cope with their fears.

Most people need their physical, emotional, spiritual and information needs identified and addressed as best as possible.

This is the starting point of all care. Begin with the most pressing issues. Once they are addressed you will have built a foundation of trust. If you can help someone meet their basic needs, they are more likely to let you help them with other needs.

People need practical help

We get very lofty about all the things we want to do to help those we are caring for. We sometimes lose sight of things like: doing the laundry, washing dishes, shoveling the driveway in the winter snow, cooking, cleaning, paying bills, returning correspondence, returning phone calls, running errands, feeding the pets, letting an employer know what is happening, letting other family and friends know what is happening, or planning time to sit and enjoy the warmth of the sun.

These practical things may not seem as important as resolving conflicts within a family (if that is ever possible) or preparing for discharge from a hospital back home. But all of these things are important. To know how much – just try not doing them and see what happens! The electricity is turned off, the mail isn't delivered, and Uncle Harry wonders what is happening to his sister.

Most people need loving people they already

know around them

We sometimes isolate patients from family, friends and neighbors with our policies, procedures and routines. We ask them to leave the room when we examine or provide basic personal care rather than include them (if they want) so they can learn from you and provide similar care themselves. In our desire to be helpful and 'friendly' we may exclude people who know the patient well from providing support or even being present to the person. Our need to be present may be a selfish one if it precludes others who know and love the person from being present. If our air of 'professionalism' infers that loved ones are incompetent to feed, bathe, or clothe the patient then we prevent them have having wonderful, intimate moments of profound care and love. We need to ask the patient whom they want in the room with them.

Most people need practical help with daily events and tasks

Dying does not provide an excuse to stop paying the bills, putting the garbage at the curb on pick up day nor shoveling the snow from the driveway or having the groceries stored away and cooked. All of the mundane tasks of living still require attention. Income tax returns still need to be filed, the banking needs to be done, the paper work (insurance, disability payments, notification to various agencies, correspondence, and family bookkeeping still need to get done). The person will likely have some family members deal with some of these things but may still require help from professional and volunteer care providers for other tasks.

Most people need their life valued.

People continue to need to be seen as Mary or John rather than as a patient with cancer or heart disease. This is most difficult to do when the patient:

- has disfiguring tumors,
- reminds us of a loved one who has died of a similar condition,
- is our age,
- has a condition that we would "rather be dead than have..."

As difficult as it may be, helping people to see

that they are "whole" regardless of their illness is an invaluable gift and our most powerful skill in helping them live fully until they die.

People need a safe place to die

Most people would prefer to die at home surrounded by familiar people and things. The home is where they feel safest and most under control. My mother very consciously, and with great physical effort, took one last walk around her home weeks before she died. She knew that soon she would be bedridden and not have a chance to do this so she went into every room and had a good long look and, quietly, said goodbye.

Some people, for whatever reason, cannot die at home but they still need a safe place to die. This can be in someone else's home (relative or neighbor), in a long-term care facility or in the hospital. Each place must provide the hospice palliative care philosophy of care in order to provide the person and their family with the physical, emotional, spiritual and information care they deserve. When that level of care is not possible, then the place is not safe for the patient and their family.

People need meaningful activity

Most people need meaningful activity centered mostly in typical situations rather than grouping people who are dying together.

Sometimes in our desire to help people who are dying we bring them together in a separate location to receive support, activities and comradeship with people going through similar circumstances. Often participants in these programs say this is the highlight of their week.

When we do this to the exclusion of other more typical activities we are separating them from the community within which they have always lived. Each time we introduce new people into their lives it is someone to whom they have to inevitably say goodbye. If these new people are also dying, then the goodbyes are increased dramatically. Each new visit to the group will likely involve news that someone they know has died.

That is not to say that such programs should close down. Such programs provide support to both the patient and their families but they should not be the highlight of a person's week. The highlight should be times when they are with people they already know and love and to whom they know they will have to say goodbye.

Their "free" time should also be filled surrounded by people within their own communities who they may already know and, if not, who are likely to be able to drop by for tea or a visit when they are in the neighborhood. For example, many respite or day programs offer arts and crafts and other activities. People can also be supported to go to their local community centre, art guild, hobby group, and the card-playing club that they have traditionally belonged to and used. Rather than limiting someone to bowling or mini-put in a day program at the local hospice or seniors' complex, encourage them to go to their golf club, local bowling alley or sports centre to be with others they already know. Provide them with the physical and personal support they need to feel comfortable using their own community resources.

The advantage of using local facilities is that the people who work there will become accustomed to customers who are not all healthy and well. They will learn invaluable customer service skills while family and friends, neighbors and club members learn how to be supportive to someone who is ill. Even if the person can no longer actively participate, they can still enjoy the camaraderie of being with people they know.

At some point they may well decide they do not want to participate in such activities but rather have their club members over to their home or take the opportunity to say a final 'goodbye' to them on their last outing out.

That is not to say that some people would not enjoy talking with others who are dying and to share their experiences and learn from each other. That is a more difficult goal than just ensuring they are at the day program every Tuesday afternoon. We must be thoughtful about the consequences of our care so that we do not congregate people who are dying to make our professional or volunteer work easier. If the patient definitely benefits from respite or day programs, that is wonderful. If they would rather be doing something else, try to see how their needs can be accommodated.

Most people need competent health care

I have said several times that inadequate pain and symptom control is inexcusable. Beyond that, competent health care looks at a person's other needs to ensure that they are addressed and managed as best as possible. People working in health care who are uncomfortable being with someone who is dying need either to acquire the knowledge and skills to become comfortable or ask to be assigned to other patients.

When incompetent care is given to a patient, it is up to the colleagues to advocate for the patient. We must never expect that patients and their families have the knowledge and skills to advocate well enough to get the care that they deserve. That is up to the professional care providers within the health care system. If the professionals cannot, for whatever reason, do it themselves then they must help the family speak to someone within the system who can help them.

Most people need valued social roles preserved

Everyone has fulfilled valued roles in their lifetime: as a family member, worker, leader, volunteer and friend. People can always be helped to create new valued roles as a wise person, advisor, or storyteller. Someone who feels their life has been meaningless can be helped to feel like they have had, and can still have, a valued social role worthy of their dignity. As people's energy and abilities decrease over time, they may need assistance in helping to remember their real contributions to families, friends, their community, their workplace and spiritual community. You need to be specific so that the patient understands you are not just trying to make them feel good but are actually helping them to understand the valued roles they can still fulfill within their family and community.

We must always remember that we cannot give someone dignity. It is an inherent quality so we can only help people identify the dignity they have within themselves.

Most people need control over their life and death through the palliative philosophy of care rather than the short cut of euthanasia or assisted suicide

This human need is sometimes described as the right to die with dignity versus the right to death.

Most often when someone asks for euthanasia (where someone kills them on their request) or assisted suicide (where someone helps them to kill themselves), the request is either: (a) a way to have control over their lives, or (b) a cry for help asking for someone, anyone, to help them with their physical, emotional, spiritual and information needs.

The request should never be "brushed aside." The request is real and worthy of a thoughtful response. One English hospice physician I spoke to, for example, spoke of the several hundreds of his patients with ALS (Amyotrophic Lateral Sclerosis or Lou Gehrig's disease). He said that quite a few had asked for his help to end their lives through euthanasia especially when their pain was severe upon entering the hospice or because they did not want to imagine going onto a respirator to help them with their breathing. Only one continued to request euthanasia after her pain and symptoms were well managed because of her suicidal tendencies that had existed long before her ALS. All the others stopped their request for euthanasia. For those in pain, once he had controlled it, euthanasia was no longer an issue. For those who feared a respirator, they discovered that when the time came to decide whether they wanted the respirator or not that most had a stronger will to live to be present at a special anniversary, a grandchild's graduation or wedding or the birth of a child or grandchild. Their will to live didn't diminish they fear of respirator but the physician and his staff's expertise helped them to adjust so they could continue to live fully (including travel, go on outings, having loved ones share a meal with them, and more).

Some expressed a fear of choking to death as they had heard this was common. When told that patients with ALS do not choke to death, they were skeptical. "Why have other people told me that it does happen?" The doctor explained that many family members believed that when a patient was having difficulty swallowing food, that the best thing to do was to give them soups, water and other liquids. This is, in fact, the opposite of what should happen. Liquids do not trigger the swallowing reflex. What is needed is to have food ground into a thick liquid that does trigger the swallowing reflex.

In all cases, information combined with excellent hospice palliative care ensured that the patients lived a more full life than they had expected. The request for euthanasia was answered with options that were valuing and life affirming.

That said, a request for euthanasia cannot always be so easily turned into a request for help with living. There are people who genuinely would prefer not to live and would prefer to die on their own terms and at their own time. The requests are still illegal in most jurisdictions. Part of the reason for the illegality is the practical provision of this service. In The Netherlands, for example, where euthanasia is legal, it occurs more often than reported that a person has requested to die on a certain date, their family and friends are called together at 'the end,' the physician is present and the person decides that, in fact, they feel pretty good that day and would like to reschedule. Depending on the schedules of their family, friends and the physician they may be able to postpone or they feel direct, or indirect, pressure to go ahead with the plan. This is only one practical aspect of euthanasia that cannot be dealt with by policies and procedures. There are many others. For examples, why ask physicians to be responsible for euthanasia when many of them are the reason there is a hospice movement in the first place – because they were not trained to provide excellent end-of-life care. If they cannot provide adequate pain and symptom control, why would you expect them to know when to provide euthanasia?

There are many unanswered questions about euthanasia and assisted suicide that are not covered in the public debate. We argue over the grand picture without looking at the specific details of how it might work. Why are people within the disability movement so adamant and so united in their opinion that euthanasia will increase the abuse of vulnerable people such as those who are poor, old, speak a foreign language, alone without advocates, disabled or likely to be dying sometime soon. Their many experiences with the health care system has convinced them, without doubt, that their lives are already at risk of ending prematurely. Why would they trust a system, therefore, to ensure risk-free euthanasia or assisted suicide?

This book is too short to go into all of the facets of this debate. See the Resources for further information. However, for people determined to die, your role can, legally, only be to provide them with sources of information that may help them with their decision.

Most people need hope maintained, discovered and enriched at all times during the process of living till death

If euthanasia and assisted suicide are often a cry for help, then the alternative is to help people identify their hopes and help them fulfill them in their remaining lives so they, and their families, create memories of love, togetherness and mutual understanding. This sense of hope comes from their perspective of what is important. Many people who thought they wanted to die rethink their wish when reminded of a special anniversary or birthday or other event that they wanted to attend. Hope for them may also be a desire to help prepare their family members as much as possible. My mother awoke from a coma that was expected to kill her because of a conscious choice she made to live longer. She told us she knew that my father, sister and I were not ready yet for her to die and that we needed time to prepare emotionally and spiritually for her death. She lived another three months to give us that time.

Most people need discerning people

Discerning people are perceptive, sensitive and astute in ways that help the person who is dying and their family live fully and experience all the positive aspects of this unique period in every one's life. They are strong advocates and know how to get results that meet the person's physical, emotional, spiritual and information needs. Discerning people understand the health care and hospice care systems and understand some of what is being experienced by the person who is dying. They are people who instinctively, or with training, understand the basic principles and specific skills identified in this book. They are likely people like you.

Most people need an 'asker'

A good death includes a strong, consistent advocacy role and an "asker" who gets things done.

From a group of discerning people in the patient's life, one or more need to take on the role of advocate; of the "asker" who asks for what the patient needs. This is often not the most immediate family member but someone only slightly removed but who can concentrate on this role. It might not be the patient's spouse but perhaps a knowledgeable child or family friend. In the coming years it may well be a professional advocate who specializes in helping people at the end of their lives when no one else in the patient's life can fulfill the role.

People who provide care also need to take care of themselves

It is important to recognize one principle rule: it is okay to live an unbalanced life for a short time in helping someone live fully until they die. This is especially true for family members who may not get enough sleep for weeks on end, may not eat well or exercise as much as they usually do. Their time is short with their loved one and if they need to be there rather than taking care of themselves, they should not be told to take care of themselves better. Let them follow their heart.

However, in the longer-term if they are caring for someone for months or if you are caring for people as part of your career, then you must take care of yourself. You are the role model for the others providing care. You are the role model for your own family and friends. Hospice care teaches us to nurture relationships above all else – we cannot do that we are not taking care of ourselves. Get whatever support or professional assistance you need to eat well, exercise often, sleep enough and balance your home and work life appropriately. You do not have to give up your own family in order to support patients and their families. You may need to help your organizations recruit more people to share the load and advocate for more resources to cover the costs.

In meeting people's needs you will need to fight for them systemically. Health care often feels like a 'fight' for patients and their families. They cannot fight for themselves because they are exhausted, overwhelmed and often frightened. They need advocates that will change the whole system.

If people within your community hesitate to provide the needed resources remind them that they will be in a similar situation soon with their own loved ones. No one escapes this inevitable ending yet many decision makers act as if patients belong to the "them" category while health care providers are the "us." We all deserve to get the support that we expect to receive ourselves – every last one of us. Never fight alone – find allies and work together to make a difference – one person at a time.

See chapter on *Care for the Caregiver* for more details.

UNDERSTANDING GRIEF

We all experience grief from the time we are young children. We all learn from grief. We all help, or hurt, others with their grief depending on how we deal with our own. Grieving is a spiritual, physical and emotional journey that both patients and families experience. How you dealt with past grief is a strong predictor of how you deal with the next one.

Simply put, grieving is emotionally, physically and spiritually painful. It opens us up to our deepest feelings of love, anger, joy, rejection, compassion, loneliness, wholeness and fear. We might grieve intensely for weeks, months or for years. Over time our days of grieving turn into hours of grieving and then, perhaps, only minutes of grieving. However, no matter how long our periods of grief, it can be just as intense as the day the person we love died. A song on the radio, a smell of familiar perfume on the street, a dream or a special anniversary can all bring back intense grief. The difference is that it might only last a few seconds or minutes rather than days.

Grieving is a natural process. It is the price we pay for deep love. Sometime the price feels overwhelming. We may have physical symptoms like tightness in our chest or our throats, trouble breathing or a choking sensation. We may feel empty in our stomach and heart. We may want to sleep for days or we cannot sleep well at all. We may not want to eat, become easily distracted and forgetful, and feel anxious or irritable. Some people become depressed, feel isolated or feel overwhelming guilt. These are all fairly typical feelings. As overwhelming as it may seem, we survive, heal somewhat and continue to live. At first it may be very hard just to get out of bed and have breakfast. Over time, we can do more and feel the hurt for shorter periods of time. With effort over many months, or perhaps years, we become stronger for the experience. Later in the chapter, I present some specific ideas that have helped many other people deal with their grief.

Grieving does not go through 'stages.' There are no stages of denial, anger, depression, bargaining with God and finally acceptance. A chaplain dealing with the feelings of people surviving cancer originally wrote these stages. Dr. Kubler-Ross added to this information and created a list of 13 stages for people who were dying. However, she later reminded people that people do not go through these stages sequentially but experience some or all of these negative (as well as positive feelings) in different orders and at different times.

If you have ever 'lost' a child in a supermarket only to find them two aisles over you will know what it feels like to go from complete relief, to overwhelming anger to genuine love for your child – all within seconds! You might have said to them: "Thank God I found you and if you ever do that again, I'll kill you!" So great was your relief. Grieving is similar in that you can go from one emotion (positive or negative) to the next one and back again within seconds. There is no logical sequence other than the sequence you might typically follow when you are grieving or very sad.

We do not wish grief on anyone, yet we all learn from our grief. Grief can make us stronger and can make us better children, spouses, parents, friends and neighbors. Grief can also make us weaker when it overpowers our ability to cope with day-to-day activities over long periods of time.

There is no right or wrong way to grieve unless your grief continues to harm you, and others, long after a loved one has died.

How we grieve depends on our cultural and personal experiences with other grief. Grief may come to us after we fail an important exam, or lose a job, or move to a new home, or break up with our first boyfriend or girlfriend. Each time we experience grief we set a pattern of how we deal with future grief. We can change how we grieve over time but it takes a conscious and ongoing effort.

Grieving is often called 'work' and a 'journey'. It takes effort and time to move from the initial grief after someone's death to when the grief is something you can live with in a healthy way; finding new ways to live without the person we miss.

At some unique point for you, you can have a new relationship with the person who has died, make new commitments to others and enjoy love in new ways.

You know when your grieving journey is at a more comfortable point when you can miss someone without being sad that they are not there. When we are in the middle of intense grief there is no difference between missing someone and being sad. At some point, you can wish that someone were here with you at a wedding, a birth, or a special family dinner without feeling sad that they are not there. The memories of them are more comforting than sad. For some people this point comes after several months of grieving. For many of us, however, this point might take a few years. There will probably, always be some times when missing someone and being sad they are not here become one feeling again. At these times, the intensity of grief might be the same as when the person died, but the duration of that intense grief lasts for minutes rather than days.

People who die continue to help the living. Not in material or even mystical ways but because they influenced our lives through the life they lived. The lessons and example they gave us continue to influence our thoughts and the way we view the world. When we have a hard decision to make we think how they might have handled it. If our relationship with them was mostly positive, we try to do things in similar ways as they did. If our experiences were mostly negative, we use their lessons as examples of what not to do. No matter our history with the person, they continue to teach us.

To reach that place of greater comfort we must go through difficult and painful events like funeral preparations, cleaning out closets, finding and reading old letters, getting through the bureaucratic paper work to settle the estate and more. Each painful event is part of the healing process although it might not feel very healing at the time.

THOUGHTS ABOUT GRIEVING

Grieving may begin weeks or months before someone dies. This is called anticipatory grief because we anticipate a life without our loved one. This grief may have its ups and downs as you experience the ups and downs of someone's illness. One day the person may feel quite good and energized so anticipatory grief may be less. If there is a sudden deterioration in their condition, your grief might be greater.

A common occurrence in anticipatory grief happens when a person is near the end of their life and death is expected soon. My mother had cancer throughout her body. One day she went into an unexpected coma from which she was not expected to wake up. For several days, we all prayed for a peaceful end to her life. During this time I went to a funeral home to arrange her funeral so that we would not have to make rush decisions after her death. When I returned from the funeral home I was told that my mother had woken up and wanted to see me. One minute I was praying for her peaceful death and grieving my upcoming loss; the next minute I was praying for her to live longer. Such a roller coaster is painful as it calls into question what we should be praying for and how best we can help each other during such difficult times. My mother lived another three months.

Another time when the grieving process can be very difficult is when family members keep a vigil for days on end only to have the patient die in the few minutes that the family are out of the room to speak with a doctor, get a cup of coffee or have a quick shower. The sense of guilt for leaving their loved one alone compounds the grief dramatically. I remind people, however, how difficult it can be to die when the people you love most are in the room with you watching you breathe and waiting for you to die.

When my mother was in her last weeks and in a semi-coma most of the time, we could no longer keep awake day and night. We brought in a night nurse who was a wonderful gift to my mother and our family. My father recognized how difficult it might be for my mother to die so he told her one night (soon after my parents' anniversary and my sister's birthday) that it would be okay for her to let go whenever she was ready. We kissed her good-night and went for some much needed sleep. Within an hour the nurse called us to be with my mother for her last few minutes. Although her death was very difficult for us we knew that she left without worrying about us as she had done three months before when she forced herself awake from a coma because we were not ready for her death yet.

Lastly, grief can be compounded in the last days by not knowing that people often stop breathing for up to two minutes or more and then start to breathe again. We did not know this so when my mother stopped breathing, we thought she had died. To have her start breathing again was terrible shocking and we thought we were doing something wrong. I now tell people that this is quite common and not to rush to any decisions about when someone dies. Let nature take its course and remain quiet during these last moments. There is no rush to call the funeral home or family doctor. You can wait hours before you make those calls so do not worry about "doing" anything. Rather concentrate on "being with" the person you love and the rest of your family.

The following tips may help you help those who are grieving, including yourself.

Feel your hurt rather than fighting it or masking it with medication or alcohol. If you do not take the time to experience the pain of grief now it will remain inside you until, perhaps, another tragedy overwhelms you. You may see people grieve over the death of a pet with such force and drama that you wonder if they are sane. It may be that they are reliving previous, unresolved grief. Grief needs to be experienced but some people can live their whole lives without going through the complete grief process. Their ability, however, to love fully and live enthusiastically may also be affected.

Experiencing grief may feel like the world is coming to an end. It is physically and emotionally painful. Sharing this feeling with others who understand grief can be helpful but it will not instantly take the pain away. Only time, supportive family and friends and lots of time spent thinking, feeling, talking and reflecting on experiences will work. Some people look inward through prayer or meditation for peace and a bigger perspective of how grief can help them. Others look outward to see how they might help others in the neighborhood, in their spiritual community or through volunteer work.

Knowing that this debilitating sense of loss is normal and that it becomes less difficult to deal with over time may help you to make it through this process as a whole person.

It is not easy for most of us. Some people may harbor real, intense grief for decades. Some people do die of a 'broken heart' after someone they loved beyond words has died. I suspect that my father died of a broken heart even though the death certificate says emphysema and brain tumors.

The death of a child or the death of a loved one who died because of violence can be the most difficult to deal with for some people. Others may see these people as 'coping very well with day-to-day life'. They may, however, never be able to love and commit themselves to others in the same way as they did before. If they accept help through professional counseling or through their spiritual leaders, they may heal part of this deep wound. Sharing their stories with people who have had similar situations can also be very helpful.

Your emotions may include feelings that you think are unhealthy or abnormal. Some people feel a strong relief that the person has died. If the person had wanted to die or if the family has provided care for a long time, relief is quite a typical feeling. Your life has been on hold for a time and now it can continue in new ways.

Regret and guilt are also common feelings. You wish that you had said or done something before the person died or feel guilty that you did something wrong. Regret and guilt are powerful emotions that take time to heal, if they ever do. The healing comes through understanding that all of us have regrets and feelings of guilt. We can either do something about our feelings or let them simmer. Some people, for example, wished that they had expressed their love more to someone who died. They might express that love at a graveside or through art or music. Or they might use the experience to express their feelings more often with the people still in their lives now.

There may be times, such as at a funeral, a social gathering, or at work when you get a sense of the world being unreal – almost as if you were watching yourself in a film. The experience of death and dying can be so intense that the only way to cope is to, quite naturally, distance yourself from the feelings for a time. A young boy whose father died in a corporate jet refused to admit that his father had died. Instead, he told people that his father was a spy and was just on a secret mission. Through the prodding of a counselor who was trying to help him understand 'the truth' he finally burst out with: "I know he's dead. I'm just not ready yet." The story/ fantasy was his way of making his world unreal for a time until he was ready to deal with his father's death. He was taking care of himself in the best way he knew how. He needed support more than confrontation – acceptance more than well-intended truth.

Face the reality of the death. Begin by continuing small daily activities, return to work when you feel ready (although employers and society may only give you five days of bereavement leave – we must change this!), continue your relationships with people you are close to, and talk about your feelings when you can.

The reality of death may hit hardest when you begin to clean out the person's closet, collect their things and perhaps, give some of them away. There is no need to do this within the first few days or weeks after someone's death. Take your time. People who have rushed through their home to clear out the person's effects days after a death have told me years later that they wished they had taken more time. Death seems so unreal around the time of a funeral and the days right afterwards. Wait before hurrying to 'tidy things up'. The same advice is true for moving away from a home shared with the person who has died. Again, there is no hurry. If you plan to move, take some time to say goodbye to the memories of that home before creating memories in a new home.

Remember the good and the bad. The person who died was not an angel or a devil. They were human. Talk to someone about these memories. You may want to repeat over and over again what your feelings are and what memories you have that are important. Find some friends to talk or write to about these feelings. Repetition is important to make your loss real. Tell them what you need and ask if they will help you.

Seek spiritual help. Ask for support, guidance and mutual prayer from members of your spiritual community, whether through a specific faith community or through family and friends who share a spiritual belief with you. Walks through nature can be very spiritual. Time meditating can help. Listening to inspirational music and reading spiritual books can be comforting.

External supports. If you rely on books for comfort, then begin to read again. If travel or work is therapeutic then do that. If you need to hide away for a few days to allow yourself to feel depressed, then give yourself that time. Playing a musical instrument or singing vigorously may be therapeutic.

When you feel ready, begin to invest your emotional energy in new relationships or stronger relationships with old friends. It is not a betrayal of the person who has died or an effort to forget him. It is sharing your love again as you did with the person who has died.

Write a journal of your feelings or write letters to the person who has died with any thoughts and feelings you feel were not said to the person when they were alive. Writing or recording one's feelings and ideas can be very healing. Writing to a close friend is another wonderful way to get the jumble of thoughts out of your head and onto paper. It helps people to think more clearly.

Past grief can help you now. For most of us, we have memories of going through very difficult situations and coming out of that experience to continue to enjoy our lives. Even when your body and heart do not feel like those good feelings will return, allow your mind to remember past experiences with grief and the joys and love you have experienced since then. This won't speed up your grieving or relieve the pain. Overcoming past grief, however, will provide that light at the end of the tunnel. There is much love, gratitude and service ahead of you when you are ready.

People who are dying may have different emotions or they may keep denying their illness to the end. People who are grieving may do the same by denying their need to experience grief. At the same time, not all of their anger or depression is caused by their grief. Their life continues and so do normal frustrations with plumbing, rude drivers, and job tensions. If you understand whether your own feelings are from grief or from normal living you can accept the reality of your situation and deal with your stresses more realistically.

My parents and grandfather died within four years of each other. I cared for all three in their homes until they died. My father was the last to become ill. After my mother and grandfather had died, I felt their loss very deeply and for a long time. What I had failed to learn through both periods of grief was that in concentrating on my grief I was missing opportunities to become even closer with my father and friends. I was feeling more inward. When my father became ill I recognized that I had missed chances to be fully with him. I wouldn't have had to deny my grief but I could have taken more 'breaks' from it to be more fully with him.

In other periods of grief since then I have not made the same mistake. When my father died I made sure to nurture the relationships closest to me. I did not turn inward all the time. I reached out, shared my feelings and tried to create happy memories with those still alive.

When trying to help a friend or family member deal with their grief, it is important to listen to their stories, their feelings and their concerns. You may hear these ideas from them over and over again during months of conversations. At some point, however, perhaps many months after a person's death, just listening to a grieving friend's stories is not enough. People must move beyond their feelings. Sometimes they use us to postpone their inevitable need to move on. We can hold them back by being too supportive. This is a hard distinction to make but it is important. If a friend cannot move on with their life and continues to hurt themselves by wallowing in grief, then, as a friend, you need to help them see what is happening. The only way it may work is to refuse to listen to the old stories without the person also talking about what they are going to do to help themselves work through the grief. This is a most difficult situation to be in but as a friend, you must be the stronger character rather than the excuse. How to know when the time has come to change the type of support you offer? You might ask yourself, "How has my friend's grief changed in six months, if at all? How must it change so that I can continue to be supportive?"

CHILDREN'S GRIEF

A child's first experience with the death of a loved one is very difficult. They have no real comparison to make with previous grief. The death of a gold fish or other pet may help them draw some comparisons but the intensity is quite different.

We do not know how to deal with children's grief. It is not part of our education. We are often uncomfortable just talking about death generally, never mind helping a child who has lost someone very important in their lives. There are books, videos and organizations such as *The Childhood Cancer Foundation – Candlelighters Canada* and *Bereaved Families of Ontario* that have a vast store of information and services that can help. The following information barely touches on some of the major issues.

We often underestimate a child's grief because they do not easily talk about their confusing feelings. They do not know what 'normal' is and may be afraid to admit to feelings of real fear of abandonment, despair, anger, guilt, loss or confusion. Death is difficult to understand at any age. It is about 'forever' and the person never coming back to us. Children need to understand these concepts but that takes time and experience. Talking is not always the way they will learn these ideas. They may lack the maturity or concentration to understand fully what the death of a loved one means to them. Younger children are in the 'here and now' in most of their activities while adults tend to focus 'way back' and 'far ahead'.

Children need your example to understand what are typical feelings and how to deal with them. They need to see the adults in their lives expressing sadness, confusion and uncertainty. They also need to see adults go on with their lives in ways that encourage the child to understand that even in tragedy, one can move forward.

One way to prepare for the death of a loved one is to encourage a child to do special things with that person or to create something special to give to the person. Any positive memories of time spent together or time spent making something for the person can add courage and strength during the grieving process. After a death, a memory book or collection of items can be made to celebrate the life shared with the loved one. For some children, making or choosing something special to include in the casket or to give other family members at the funeral can be comforting.

Many children need the reassurance that they are not at fault for the death. They may remember saying something, like "I wish you were dead," or "I'm going to kill you" as part of a game they were playing or out of anger to the person who died. They may feel that if they had done or said something they could have prevented the death. Understanding how the person really died reassures them that they are not responsible.

Children also worry about themselves. If Grandma or Dad has died, what will happen if the other adults taking care of them die? They may worry about being abandoned and need reassurance that they will always be well cared for in any circumstance. Again, helping them see what really caused the death and that other adults in their life right now do not have a similar disease or condition can help. Reassurance and love are always better than a quick "You don't have to worry dear."

It is not helpful insisting that a child talk about death. However, every question should be answered. Take advantage of opportunities to talk about death. For example, news reports of a death, a neighbor's death, or a program on television may help you discuss the child's feelings. We cannot make it 'okay' for children within days of a death in the family. It will take them many months and years, just as for their parents, to come to terms with all the aspects of someone's death. Do not rush them.

Children are not adults. They need to be children. If a parent has died, the child should not be expected to become the 'man' or 'woman' of the house. The remaining adults may need extra supports, but it should not be the children who provide that adult support. Children can be wonderfully supportive as children but they should not fulfill the role of the adult who has died.

When children ask questions that you have no answer for, say so. "I don't know" is a wonderful phrase because it means that the adult and child can look for answers together. Some questions, of course, have no answers and that is part of life too. Children can often tell when someone has told them something that is untrue, too simplistic or gives a quick answer to keep them from asking more questions. If children feel this happening often, they will shut out the adults and withdraw or act out in frustration or anger.

Children need the security that comes from rituals, rules and structure. They need limits and consistent discipline that tells them they are loved, safe and part of a family that works things out together. If parents are having trouble providing these things during difficult times, they must look for outside help to give their children and themselves comfort and support.

Children have wisdom that is often overlooked. They may want to save items of personal importance from the person who has died. They may want to create a scrapbook of pictures, artwork, poems and thoughts. They recognize, intuitively, that collecting memories is a way to deal with grief. Encourage their natural tendencies and ask them to explain why they have chosen certain items over other ones. You may be surprised by the depth of their thinking and comforted by their genuine love.

Children may have temporary periods of needing to hold onto to their parents or a trusted adult for comfort. They might have nightmares or wet their beds. These 'regressions' are just a sign that they need extra caring and time with trusted adults. My grandfather was 92 when he was dying and he spoke of wishing that his mother were there to hold him. We never lose that desire to be safely in the arms of someone we trust. Children express this need more through actions than words and we must pay attention. They also have short attention spans so you may see them laughing and playing soon after a death or at the funeral. Young children may appear to forget that someone they love has died but they are actually just being children. They will come back to their feelings and questions over the months and years ahead. We must be patient and understanding of their different ways of coping with difficult, emotional times.

ELDERS' GRIEF

Our elders have experienced grief many times. If they experienced the horrors of war, the Depression years, or the death of a child, grandchild or spouse, they have dealt with grief in ways that many people cannot imagine. Their longevity probably means that they also have dealt with the grief of losing many friends, co-workers and acquaintances. They probably are also grieving the loss of some of their physical and mental abilities. Grief is a constant companion for many of them. As they anticipate their own deaths, they deal with the grief of saying goodbye to loved ones left behind.

At the same time, their experiences have given many of them an understanding of grief, of their own responses to grief and how best they can be supported and supportive. Elders have, through longevity and experience, much to teach younger people about coping with the difficulties of life. They can show great empathy to a young mother whose husband has died. They can understand the trauma of their grandchildren as they begin to explore the world of relationships, study and work. That same empathy is possible in reverse as grandchildren, family and friends can empathize with part of their elders' grief when a spouse, friend or family member dies. When my grandfather was dying, he spoke about feeling like an orphan without his mother there to comfort him. He was 92 years old and he missed his mother as I did mine. We have much more in common with our elders than we sometimes realize.

Elders are no more perfect or ideal than younger people. They can be angry, lonely or unkind at times like everyone else. They do, however, offer a wealth of knowledge and skills. This offer is not always accepted by those around them and in North America, we have tended to isolate them from their communities.

In helping an elder deal with grief, it might be best to allow them to 'teach' us about grief from their perspective. In listening to their lessons we might find ways to be most helpful. It is also important to recognize that the person within an older body still feels many of the same emotions that younger people do. A friend of mine was once talking about the old people in the seniors' home where she lived. I asked her how old those people were. "Oh in their seventies or early eighties, I guess," she replied. "Are you old," I asked her. "Heavens no, dear." She was 86 and felt much younger because her interests had not changed very much over the decades. My grandfather still had a glint in his eye when he told us about putting a girl's ponytail in the ink well in 1899. He still had some of the mischievous personality of a 10-year-old boy at 92 years of age.

SPECIAL EVENTS

Special holidays or events may trigger difficult

emotions. After my mother died I often wished that she could be with us for Christmas, holidays, birthdays and other special events. It was not until my father died four years later that I understood that my spending so much time wishing my mother was at certain events, meant I did not pay enough attention to my father who was there.

Many people have more difficulty in the days before a special event than the day itself. In our anticipation of a difficult day we actually lessen the effect of the day itself.

Here are a few tips for dealing with special days:

- Get extra support from family and friends. If you choose to be alone for that day, purposefully mix feelings of happy memories with sad ones. We need to remember the good and the bad of such events and use these lessons to help us cope. If you over-indulge in food or drink, recognize that you don't want to do that every day or else you will hurt yourself. Feel the emotions that are there. Sob if you need to. Laugh if you want to. There are no rules about what you MUST do, only suggestions about what you might do to help yourself and others that are grieving too.

- Make lists if you have trouble around such events remembering simple chores, gifts to buy, places to be on certain days, or cards to mail. On the list, mark off any items that are important to do first. Lists give us some sense of control and satisfaction as well tick off items that we complete.
- Some traditions you will want to keep and others you may want to change. You will get lots of free advice from caring family and friends. Go with your instincts as long as they do not hurt others. For example, you may not have liked a certain dish that was prepared for every formal family event. You will not dishonor the person's memory by choosing to cook something else.
- Some people spend money to 'take the pain away'. An elaborate vacation, too much shopping or too many dinners away from home will hurt you financially. Don't spend your way through grief as it only adds the grief of financial troubles. You may inherit money after the death of a loved one. Take some time before spending any of it. You have a whole life ahead of you and your

loved one was trying to help you by easing your financial burdens.

- You may get many invitations to parties, get-togethers, and special events. People may want you to attend to 'take your mind off things' when that is not what you want to do. They may worry that you are too isolated on your own. You need to judge at what point you are ready to socialize. These events are usually not the time or place to talk about your grief so you may not want to attend soon after a death. Instead, you might invite people over for informal visits to chat or ask someone to go for a walk with you. People mean well but you must decide when the time is right. On the other hand, do not isolate yourself from those who care about you. Find other ways to spend time with them. If you do not, they may well stop asking to be with you and your isolation from people who care about you may become permanent.
- New rituals can help ease grief. Lighting a candle to honor the life of a loved one is an age-old tradition. Playing favorite music or watching a favorite film can bring back happy memories.

These memories may also bring sadness. Feel the emotions that come. Purposely balance the happy and sad feelings you have.

- On the anniversary date of the person's death, you might decide to create a new ritual of celebration to honor the person's life and their importance in your life. It might be as simple as a visit to the cemetery or going for a walk in your favorite spot together. It might be reading a special book or writing to loved ones to share the love you had with the person who died.

Feel the feelings at appropriate times. Remember the good and the bad memories. Use what you have learned to help others. At least, that is what so many others do, with perfectly human, mixed results. We can only do the best we can do, day-to-day, month-to-month and year-to-year. What a gift our experiences can be to others.

CHAPTER 5

Practical Knowledge for Caregivers

You know most of the following. They are in no particular order. The question is, do you use these ideas? Do you teach them? Do you role model them to others? Do you do these things instinctively or consciously and thoughtfully? Do you make the effort to demonstrate many of these ideas to family members so they, too, can use them? Do you use these ideas consistently or only as you remember them?

Note: some of the following tips are more appropriate for professional and volunteer caregivers while others are more helpful for family and friends.

1. Remember that **care giving is mutual**. It is not better to give than to receive. When

you recognize the equality of caregiving and receiving care, you enter in the realm of true love and compassion. You will be a real person again rather than a caregiver or server. You can find that well of true love that you have shared before the person's illness. You can find that balance between love, gratitude and service that is so fulfilling.

2. The **more connected you are** to your own family, friends, neighbors, colleagues from work, your community and your cultural and spiritual community, the better you will be able to deal with the ups and downs of caring for others who are dying. The nurse who cared for my mother in her last week of life was so isolated herself that when she became ill a few years later she chose suicide over the type of care she so admirably gave others.
3. We **hear only about 20%** of what someone says and forget about 80% of that within one day. That leaves us remembering only about 4% of our conversations. How much information a person can comprehend is based on this rule. If the information is

important enough it must be given in several ways at several times. Use as many of the following methods of providing information as possible to reinforce what is important. Do it gradually or all at once, whichever the person wants, to give them control over timing and volume:

> verbal conversations; written materials (books, pamphlets, articles, magazines, newsletters); DVDs and CD ROMS of facts, feelings and similar situations experienced by others including films and music; mentor/group supports; theatre; and web site links.

4. Open-ended questions + active listening + reading body language + silence = **your most powerful communication tool**. Active listening is a skill that involves listening to what a person says while also questioning what they might not be saying, and why. Active listening also involves looking at the person's body language to see if what they are saying is consistent with how they look. You can always tell when people are NOT practicing active

listening. If there is no silence in a conversation then people are thinking up their own replies to someone's comments while the other person is still talking. This is not active listening. A good listener uses the silence after someone finishes talking to think about what was said and, perhaps, rehearse what they want to reply.

When my father was dying I asked him one day what it was that was making him unhappy. Then I kept quiet. His first response was "If you were dying son, you wouldn't be too happy either." I agreed but said that what made me unhappy might be different than what was making him unhappy. I kept quiet again. He spent several minutes: (1) deciding whether he would tell me anything? (2) if so, how much? and (3) rehearsing in his mind what he would say.

When he was ready, he told me what was making him unhappy. It was not what I expected. I expected that it was because he had been forced to retire early or that he really missed my mother who had died only four years before. What was really making him unhappy was that he would not live long enough to be at my wedding.

We had discussed moving the wedding date and location so that he could attend but he had refused because it would inconvenience my fiancee's family on the west coast. He said he was happy to be with us now and not to worry. So we thought that concern was over when in fact it was not. An open-ended question + silence + watching his body language helped us to open up the discussions again so that he became more involved in the planning of the wedding.

He helped pick out music and dictated a wedding card to my sister who gave me the card the night before my wedding, six months after my father died. What a powerful gift. Just what a needed to enjoy the most important day of my life.

5. **Take care of yourself** physically, emotionally and spiritually. That means that you need to eat more healthy food and healthy drinks than junk. Pray or meditate to feel the comfort that this gives you. Take some time for a

quick walk around the block or some other light exercise. Sleep as much of a normal sleep as you can. Get others to give you extra time for 'cat naps'.

6. **When you allow a patient's family to watch you do your work**, you provide them with a role model and also a free lesson on how to provide care when you are not around. For example, when my mother came home from the hospital for her last months of life, my father and I were expected to care for her. In the hospital we were always asked to leave the room when any personal care was provided to my mother. This meant that when we needed to give my mother her first bed bath at home we were completely ignorant of how to do it properly. I asked my father, "How do you think we should do this?" He said, "It can't be that hard. I used to give you kids a bed bath when you were babies." That should have been our first clue that this was not going to go well!

   Of course we could have asked my mother how it was done but she was weak and we didn't want to bother her. She could also, of course, have told us but she did not want to make us feel ignorant so she went along for the experience. For those of you who are nurses or have given bed baths, you will understand immediately what we did wrong. For the rest of you, you get to learn from our mistakes!

My father and I got all the things we needed for the bath and proceed to undress my mother and wash her from top to bottom. Then we dried her from top to bottom. This was mid-winter in a 15th floor apartment with drafty windows. The goose bumps on my mother's skin told us she was cold from the experience but we didn't know how else to do it.

The next day a visiting home nurse arrived to provide my mother's care. She asked how our first bed bath had gone the day before and after she heard what we had done, she smiled ever so gently and suggested that we come and watch her give a bed bath. What she did was so logical, in hindsight. She never told us we had done a poor job the day before but her demonstration showed us how we would do it better next time.

She kept my mother covered with a sheet and blanket and only washed and then dried parts of my mother's body – for example, one hand at a time, then one arm at a time, then the legs, the torso, and her face. At each step, she would pull the blanket back for only a short time and after drying her with a warm towel (a few seconds in the dryer to heat it up) would cover her up again. My mother never got cold and we learned an invaluable lesson. If you work in a hospital or in home care, always encourage family members who want to, to stay and help you provide personal care. That is how we learn what to do when you are not there.

7. Consider having **a support circle.** These circles can share the work of meeting someone's physical, emotional, spiritual and information needs. Some of the circle members can provide personal care. Others can help with the grocery shopping and other household needs. Others can help with the legal and financial

issues that need to be done. One or two of the people can become the circle coordinators to make sure people do not all arrive all at once on one day and no one shows up the next. See *Family Hospice Care* or *Caring for Loved Ones at Home* for specifics of setting up such a circle.

8. **Give 'bad news'** by allowing the person to choose when to hear the news. For example, ask them if they would like it now, later today or tomorrow. This sense of control will help the patient/family very much.

   I asked my father's physician if I could be the one to tell him that he had a terminal illness. I went to my father and said, "I've spoken to your doctors and did some research into your condition. Would you like to know what I found out?"

   By giving him control over the timing of the information he also had better control over how to respond and cope with the news. He knew that if my information was 'good news' that I would have just told him. By giving him the choice of when to hear the news and how much of it at any time, he had, for the first time, control over his medical information. He took a few minutes (a long time to be quiet) to think about his answer. Finally he said, "Yes I would like to know but not right now." He could have had the news then, later or decided that he did not want it at all but for me to share it with other family members.

The next day he asked me if he would likely be alive for my wedding in June and this was September. I said it was not likely. That was all he wanted to know. The next day he asked if he would likely be alive for Christmas. I said that was unlikely too. Over the next few days he continued to ask more questions until he knew everything he wanted to know. He had total control over the flow of information.

From my standpoint, his control relieved me of the burden of figuring out when the "right time" was to tell him the news. When I teach this skill to new physicians they often say they do not have time to wait for the patient to decide when to receive the information. I suggest they still give the patient 3 options. Something like, "Mr. van Bommel. I have some news about your condition. Would you like me to tell you now, at the end of my rounds in about an hour or tomorrow morning?" These choices still would have given my father some control over his information. Few medical decisions need to be made right away. We usually have time to give people some control over their 'news.'

9. Families and volunteers need to **get as much information** as they need to provide the care they want to give, how they can do it well and where they can turn for more help. Practical advice is available in books like *Caring for Loved Ones at Home*.

10. In periods of **overwhelming stress**, you might find it helpful to concentrate and recite (silently or out loud) a quote or prayer.

   At one point in caring for my mother, I did not think I could go on. She was throwing up and all I could do was hold the vomit tray and help as best I could. I thought I was going to be physically ill myself or faint. I remembered a paraphrased version of a verse from the Bible and I kept repeating it over and over again to focus me on helping her rather than becoming sick myself. The verse helped me concentrate on something other than my fear. The verse as I remembered it from John 14:27 was, *Peace I give you, my peace I give unto you: not as the world giveth, give I unto you. Let not your heart be weary, neither let it be afraid.* Your own religious or poetic background may help you find a similar quote or prayer.

For beginning professionals, volunteers and family members this is a handy little aid. I have found this immensely helpful. Others might want to sing a song in their mind or quote a favorite poem. Whatever you can do to distract your gag reflex while still be supportive to the person you are caring for.

11. There are some **mistaken ideas** about the kind of person you need to be to care for someone:

- ***You need unlimited energy.*** Not possible so understand the need to have balance in your life.
- ***You have to accept all the responsibilities on your own shoulders.*** Heroes only survive in movies. In real life you need to share the

responsibilities whether you are a physician, nurse, volunteer or spouse of the person who is ill.

- ***If you look after yourself, you are selfish.*** How little we must think of the person who is ill to think that they do not care about our well being. If you do not take care of yourself you will probably make the person who is ill feel worse about their situation. This is a mutual experience and everyone must help each other and themselves stay as healthy and comfortable as possible. It is not better to give than to receive. Do not fall into this trap. It will hurt you, your family and your patient. Ask for and accept help.
- ***If you are exhausted, you must really care about the person who is ill.*** This is one of my favorite mistaken beliefs. I have sat in on family caregiver support groups and heard the following type of conversation more than once:

"I'm so tired today. I only got 4 hours of sleep last night."

"You got 4 hours? I would kill to have 4 hours sleep. I only had 2 hours and that was broken up several times by

my husband waking up needing help."

"You had 2 hours of sleep? I wish I knew what sleep was. I'm sure I haven't had 2 hours sleep in the past 3 days."

It almost sounds like a competition doesn't it? It is as if they were competing to see who loved their family member more and, therefore, would sacrifice more for them. It is a little like the story you might have heard growing up about how your parent or grandparent went to school barefoot in the snow, up hill both ways, for 5 miles!

Exhaustion is not a sign of love. It is a sign of neglect. You are neglecting your own health and the health of the person you are caring for. You may be more tired than usual during particularly difficult times, but then it is time to catch up. Plan to take some time off (often called respite care). It may mean taking a few days off from caregiving. It may mean the person you are caring for agrees to have a hospice or respite program provide extra home care support for a few days while you rest at a friend's home. When my grandfather was ill, I took a few days to travel to my niece's baptism. It wasn't easy leaving him (for either of us) but we knew it was necessary and my niece and I now have a lifelong memory to share of that important event.

- ***People should know what we need and offer it to us.*** This is a little like people should be able to read our minds so we don't have to think out loud. It is not going to happen. The gift of care requires more open communication than usually occurs between people. People have to discuss personal, intimate details of their lives in order to get the help they need. They need to talk about sex, or the lack of sex. They need to talk about whether they can drink alcohol or still smoke. They need to be able to ask for a cuddle or hug, not not. They need to talk about incontinence or about family difficulties. To expect people to figure it out for themselves, however, is unfair. Therefore, again, you have the opportunity to role model clear and concise communication skills that family members can learn from and copy.

- ***God will take care of you.*** There are more than a few professional and volunteer care providers who think that God will take care of them so well that they do not have to worry about good nutrition, sleep, exercise and nurturing valuable relationships. When they see it written out in black and white, of course, they recognize the fallacy of their belief but they may still need reminding every so often. God will help you spiritually and emotionally. At the same time you need to help yourself. Get support from family, friends, special groups, telephone calls with loved ones far away, moderate exercise, massage, books, good nutrition (and some special treats that may not be on the nutritionists' top ten list!), some time away for a night or two rest (called respite care), some fun everyday, writing a journal or diary, sleeping a little more, a walk in nature, reading a good book, some calming music, silence and a talk with a favorite pet. Most of these things do not have to take a lot of time but all of them will help give you an extra bit of energy. This is not selfish; it really is about meeting the loving needs of the person you are caring for and some of your own needs as well.

- ***Don't spend a lot of time thinking about your feelings.*** People believe that to be a professional requires a distance between their emotions and their work. They believe that to show their feelings or to think about their own feelings such as grief after a death is unprofessional. The reverse is true. One nurse I knew, for example, never showed grief at the death of any of her patients or even her family members. When her cat died, however, she took a week off and did nothing but cry for the week. There were so many hidden feelings. This was unhealthy and she recognized that and learned to express herself better and to think about how her work and family life are enriched when feelings are recognized and felt openly.

Our family's physician, for example, was quite angry with me because I did not invite her to my mother's funeral. I presumed that she would be too busy for such things. She was hurt and told me so. I was grateful to her because she showed genuine affection for my mother. I should not have presumed to know how she would respond to an invitation to the funeral. In fact, on the morning of my mother's death, our physician, the visiting home nurse and the home care homemaker all sat around our dining table shedding some tears and sharing stories about my mother. What a great gift they shared with us – both their time and their compassion.

12. **Torn between two or three loves** – i.e., sometimes when we try to care for someone else we lose sight of what is helpful and who else may need us. A professional or volunteer hospice care provider may be caring for their own parent who is ill while also torn between being at work where other people clearly need them and at home with their children. This most troubling dilemma must be faced squarely with the help of one's family, friends and colleagues. We cannot be all things to all people but we cannot completely isolate ourselves from others who need us even as we care for someone we truly love. Look at **support circles**

as one way to help (see *Family Hospice Care* or *Caring for Loved Ones at Home*). Some jurisdictions also offer paid compassionate leave from work to care for someone in their last weeks or months. Some organizations make it a point to recognize this "sandwich generation" by providing liberal leave benefits. The future will require even more organizations to do this as the baby boomers will require more resources than currently exist.

13. Sometimes it is necessary to **say no**. You do not need to explain why. Sometimes we feel compelled to give a long, detailed explanation of why we cannot do something. It is not necessary and often not appreciated. Whatever the reason, you are telling the person that the reason is more important than their request. Therefore, it is best to say "no" quickly and move on. That is a lot better than saying "yes" and at the last minute backing out of the agreement to help.
14. It can be very helpful to have a **private space** where you can go to hide, sleep, re-energize, pray and think. Even if it is just down the

hallway, in a hospital chapel, or a walk outside it is a special place to recover your energy and perspective.

15. **Family dynamics** cannot be understood or manipulated in the last weeks of someone's life. You cannot reconcile a family to all outstanding issues. You can help them identify behaviors and actions they can do now that can make a profound impact on the person they love. The results will benefit everyone. When they look back upon those times together they will have found memories of something special that you encouraged them to do. For example, helping loved ones write 'thank you' notes to people they love or helping them have quiet time with someone they have had difficulties with in the past. Simple acts have profound consequences. Help them identify what is possible in their specific situation. Do not live out your life's mistakes or dreams through them – concentrate on their needs.
16. **Change your time zone** to theirs. In other words, slow down your pace to match theirs as they are often concerned about the 'now'

while we are already planning months ahead. When I visit someone who is ill or grieving, I make a conscious effort outside their door to take a few seconds to slow down my breathing, take deeper breathes which also slows down my heart rate and to enter their room calm and focused just on them. I consciously push out thoughts about my next appointment, what I'm cooking that night, or what has to be picked up at the cleaners. This simple changing my pace helps the person I am visiting feel that I am there just for them and not rushed.

17. **Use direct eye contact** and a **smile** sometimes (understanding cultural differences, of course) while at other times allow the person the space not to look at you (e.g., on a walk or car ride – people may find direct eye contact too emotional). During particularly difficult discussions about grief, guilt or anger, for example, I often go for a walk with someone or sit beside them rather than across from them. This gives them control over when they want to look at me and when they want to concentrate on their own thoughts or feelings.

18. Help family members or the patient with a few of the **everyday errands**, chores and needs of their lives when you can. It may be as simple as helping them on with their coat when they are going out and you only have a few extra minutes or something more time consuming like helping them answer some mail.
19. Encourage the **recording of the person's life** in some form. See book *Recording Your Life and Family Stories* at *www.canada150.com* for instructions on how to do this.
20. **Use appropriate touch affectionately**. This is highly cultural so follow the lead of the patient. Hispanic people for example, often use touch as a common form of communication. In other cultures, such as traditional English people, touch is seen as something that is highly personal and not done in public very much.
21. Use **extra comfort measures**. For example, a warm towel given to a patient after their tub or shower; preparing their favorite dessert or hot drink, raising or lowering the temperature to their comfort level rather than keeping it at

your preferred level.

22. Use **appropriate humor, stories, and questions** to help conversations be more meaningful. Most people enjoy stories either by telling them or listening to them. Conversation is an opportunity to share such stories and increase the bond between you. As a care provider you can also demonstrate how a timely, open-ended question can open up a whole discussion about something that is quite interesting and "new" for the family too.
23. Use **people's correct names**, and help others to **remember your name**. Avoid "dear", "sweetie", and similar terms of endearment until you have earned the right to use them, if ever. Some people prefer to be called more formally by Mr. or Mrs. Browne while others prefer their first name or pet names. Ask them. Always begin with the formal until told otherwise. Terms of endearment are often an excuse not to learn the person's name.
24. **Provide distractions** (e.g., music, movies, reading material, television, activities). This can be particularly helpful if someone is

anxious, bored or lonely.

25. Take time to **leave the person** after each visit in a compassionate, unhurried way. If you have slowed down your pace before entering the person's room only to look at your watch, see that you are late and rush out of there, the whole visit feels rushed. Take the time to leave as unhurried as you arrived. The impact this will have is enormous. The person who is ill is always seeing people rush off to their interesting lives while they await their death.
26. **Help create memories** using **humor and creativity** and a conspiracy of well-meaning people to help patients, their families and other caregivers. Celebrate anything worth celebrating (birthdays, anniversaries, visits from out-of-town family and friends). Create celebrations out of nothing more than a lovely day, a favorite song heard on the radio or a bird feeding outside the person's window. Each day should have some memorable events happening that makes everyone feel special and valued. It could be as simple as holding a hand, reading a book aloud, listening quietly to music together

or sharing a special treat. These are times that force all of us to slow down from our hectic lives for a few minutes or a few hours and we should treasure each of these gifts of care.

27. **Ask people** what they want you to do to be most helpful and respectful. Of course this should be the first point in this list. However, many people do not know how to answer the question "How can I be most helpful to you right now?" With the 26 points described above, you now have a better sense of what to offer.

CHAPTER 6

Voices beyond Earshot

The following is an exercise for those of you who are professional and volunteer caregivers. Put on some quiet music as you read **aloud** the voices of your patients. You could also do this at a staff or volunteer event. Read the quotes below to your colleagues so they can learn from the voices beyond earshot.

In the hectic pace of any health care facility or in someone's home, the quiet voices of patients and families can easily be missed. These 'quotes' are distilled from conversations I have had over decades of providing care and teaching. The sentiments are real. You will be able to easily identify people you know personally and professionally who have said similar things to you. We all need to listen to these voices and share them with others so their meaning is not lost. We need to act upon these voices to help diminish fears and celebrate successes.

I'm scared. I'm so scared I may scare myself to death. Hearing myself say that sounds funny. Some people may even laugh. But newspapers are always saying how stress is a killer and I can't remember ever being this stressed. The articles also say I may get an infection and die here or that my medications may be given incorrectly. I don't know what you can do to help me with my fears – I just pray that you can think of something. I'm really, really scared.

She came out of nowhere. I didn't know her. Never been properly introduced. But there she was. She had a quiet, peaceful smile instead of one of those pasted-on smiles. She said only two words: "I know." Then she was quiet. From that moment I knew that she knew. She knew what I was feeling. She knew I wasn't sure if I would make it or not. But she knew

I would be okay – no matter what happened. Her knowing took the worst of my fears away. She just knew.

He is visiting his father next door. He smiles as he passes by. On his second visit, he smiles again and says 'hello'. On his third visit, he actually stops and asks how I am doing. I don't know him. Will never see him again after a few days. But for those few moments he saw me, recognized a fellow human being and took notice of me. His father died yesterday. He came to collect his things. I took a flower from the bouquet my daughter gave me the day before and gave it to him. I know men don't usually get flowers, but I thought he might like one anyway. He cried quietly when I gave him the flower and he nodded. We didn't need words. We were eternal friends who felt like we had always known each other. Crisis did that during the war years and it does so now too. We will always remember each other even though we never even learned each other's names.

Imagine for a moment, you are in a small theatre. The seats are full. The crowd is a buzz with anticipation. The smell of hors d'oeuvres and cheeses fill the air. The clinking of wineglasses speaks of a celebratory gathering. There is music in the air that fills your heart and lungs with energy.

You feel your heart beat racing and your breath is faster than normal. You know what is going to happen next at this theatre. You must walk onto the stage and take a bow. You take a hesitant step forward from behind the curtain. Stage fright does, surprisingly, feel a bit like what a heart attack might feel like. Yet you know you must go out onto that stage, so you do. You have always done what you needed to do.

As you hit the mark on centre stage, the spotlight is on you, and although you can no longer see the audience as you did from back stage, you know they are there because you hear thunderous applause. You sense the people are on their feet now.

The house lights come on so that you see before

you hundreds, if not thousands of people you have cared for over the years. Some patients are represented by family members as their loved ones died. Many faces you do not remember as you have cared for so many you can't possible remember them all, but they have remembered you.

A little girl comes forward and walks up the steps to present you with a huge bouquet of flowers, much as you have seen children do when Queen Elizabeth is in town. The little girl presents you the flowers and then, a little shy, but still with enough courage to complete the task, she walks up to the microphone. She unfolds a piece of paper and reads, a little too loudly at first in case the microphone does not work;

"My name is Cassandra. I have been asked by all the people you have cared for and their families to thank you for not only doing your job, but also for making us feel welcome, cared for and nurtured. You took care of my grandma last year. She died only a few months after you first met her. You did something for her that we have never seen anyone else ever do before. You saw our grandma while others saw only an old lady who couldn't remember who she was. Thank you for the gift of seeing my grandma like I saw her. You must have been someone's grandchild too once. We are all very grateful. Thank you from the bottom of our hearts."

The little girl was crying by now, and so are you and so is much of the audience. There is a human bond at the time of crisis that cannot be replicated anywhere else. You are the key to that bond happening in such a lonely place.

Whether the audience ever actually comes together in a real theatre or only in the theatre of your mind, rest assured that audience is there.

CHAPTER 7

Specific Caregiver Situations

Caring for others in such a personal and intimate way as hospice care is one of the most fulfilling and life-defining opportunities in our lives. When you care for someone else you know in your heart, mind and soul that you are making a real difference in that person's life. Caregiving gives us that unique opportunity to remember what is truly valuable in our lives and within our families and community. Caring is not always easy. It can be physically exhausting, mentally taxing and emotionally draining. It can also be exhilarating, rejuvenating, peaceful, joyful and awe inspiring.

IMMEDIATE NEEDS

When I began caring for my parents and my grandfather, I was concerned about their physical needs first and then their emotional and spiritual needs. I was not interested in people's advice that I needed to take better care of myself, get more help at home, or even that I should get back to work. I may not have been prepared for the demands of taking care of loved ones at home but I had a lifetime of preparation in a loving family to want to be with my parents and grandfather in their last months.

What other people did not understand was that I had a whole life ahead of me. Later on I could eat well, sleep longer, work and enjoy myself. Right then, I only had a few months to be with my mother, my father and my grandfather. I was not trying to be a martyr. I was not ignoring my own emotional and spiritual needs. I was fulfilling them as best I could. Taking care of my loved ones was demanding, fulfilling and terribly important to me. I did it for me as much as I did it for them. They needed me. I needed them.

Yes, I hurt myself physically by ignoring my diet, exercise and time to be alone. After my father's death I could barely move my neck for months. However, I was fulfilling one of my greatest needs to be with my parents and grandfather, revel in our love and our family history. No family is perfect. No family has perfect relationships within it. However, I would never have any of the regrets that begin with sentences like: "If only I had...." What a legacy that time together is for me. I am a better husband, father, friend and neighbor because of those intense times.

Would I do it differently today? Yes. I know more now. I can take better care of myself so that my loved ones are not as worried about me. People who are dying still worry a great deal about the people who are caring for them. By taking care of ourselves, we can minimize some of that worry.

I hope some of what I present is helpful. Do what you need to do to make this time as fulfilling and meaningful as possible. You will not have this particular opportunity again.

LONG-TERM NEEDS

Although we might hurt ourselves in short-term caregiving situations, we must be wiser when we care for someone for a long time. It might be all right to use caregiving as an excuse not to eat and drink well, exercise or sleep well. However, when you do this for any length of time you will hurt yourself dramatically and you will hurt the person you are caring for because they will worry unnecessarily.

Just as patients need support to meet their physical, emotional, spiritual, and information needs, so do family members and professional and volunteer care providers.

Knowledge and experience can deepen our reservoir of hope and courage. Eileen McArthur explains: *"As a volunteer in palliative care and later as a trainer of palliative care volunteers, I gained an understanding and a good deal of insight which served me well when I was faced with the impending deaths of my mother and my brother. My hospital experience provided me with the knowledge and experience that helped and supported both my family and me when we became the caregivers for our loved ones.*

"I saw courage, great courage, in patients and their families and I also witnessed great sadness, disappointment and guilt. I consider it a privilege to have been involved with a palliative care unit in a hospital and I know that this interest in helping to provide a 'good death' for the terminally ill will never wane."

PROFESSIONAL AND VOLUNTEER CAREGIVERS

Much of what is in this book about helping the patient and family members during a person's illness, and the grieving afterward, holds true for professional and volunteer caregivers as well. You are human beings first and some people will affect you more visibly than others. When my mother died, our family physician, the visiting nurse and the homemaker sat together and cried. They did not pretend to be strong or professionally distant. They did not worry about embarrassment and most importantly, they did not go away. They stayed and expressed their feelings honestly. It was their greatest gift to the rest of my family for it showed us their concern without words and how my mother had touched their lives.

Hospice care bereavement programs follow many of these suggestions by allowing people to express their feelings, keep in contact with some of the caregivers, and use the sense of touch to express concern.

When we look at caregiver stress, I will separate caregivers that work in palliative/hospice care from acute care doctors, nurses, therapists, clerics, psychologists and the others.

ACUTE CARE CAREGIVERS

People who work in hospitals and medical centers are used to treating patients who are there for active, cure-oriented treatment. Generally, health care systems do not provide them the time, training or staffing to provide excellent hospice care. Most give the best clinical care possible in very difficult circumstances. Some may have some of the following stresses:

- Difficulty in accepting that a patient's physical and psycho-social problems cannot always be cured or controlled.
- Difficulty in knowing when to get palliative care for their patients. In some areas, there may be little or no palliative care services available that can add to the stress.
- Difficulty in deciding how much to tell a patient about her condition.
- Difficulty in coping with the severe constraints of time and low staffing ratios involved in patient care and administrative responsibilities.
- Frustration at being involved with a patient's

family whose emotional resources have already been drained by the patient's illness.

- Disappointment at being unable to fulfill the patient or family's expectation of dying a good death.
- Depressed because they have no time to deal with their own grief when a patient is dying or has died.
- Anger at being critically reviewed by the public.
- Difficulty in deciding how involved to be with the patient and the family especially outside of normal working hours.
- Frustration in their inability to give the kind of care they want to give.
- Difficulty with their inability to be a good communicator.

PALLIATIVE/HOSPICE CAREGIVERS

The stresses of palliative/hospice caregivers differ from those of acute care staff. Although they often have more time to help patients and families, their professional position has been given less credibility because they are dealing with people who are dying. There are no miracle cures and there is an erroneous assumption that their work is, therefore, less rewarding or valuable.

With added time to spend with patients and families there are added concerns and problems to deal with. The philosophy of physical, emotional and spiritual support is not always easy to fulfill. Some patients have not accepted that they are dying. Some patients and families have major unresolved problems that frustrate the caregivers' hope for a peaceful and comforting death for a patient.

The relative newness of palliative/hospice care means that the systems have not been perfected, and may never be perfected, to everyone's satisfaction. In designing the program, frictions between well-meaning caregivers occur because each has certain beliefs about what they think is the palliative care program.

Caregivers grieve someone's death in their own individual way. In cases where they have come to know patients and their families closely, the grieving is more acute. There are few people outside of hospice care who can understand the mixture of personal satisfaction and professional stresses that these caregivers have. One of the advantages of working in hospice care is that professional stresses are more clearly identified and addressed. The following list describes some of the differences between acute care and hospice care personnel:

- There may be less conflict regarding a patient's death because hospice care is concerned with comfort rather than prolonging life.
- There may a lower patient/caregiver ratio in hospice care so that time and administrative stresses are reduced. This ratio depends on the particular hospice care model in place. Freestanding hospices and hospital units have lower staff ratios, for example but consultation teams in hospitals may not.
- There can be a team spirit in hospice care and an acceptance of the hospice care philosophy that includes more formal and informal supports for the professionals and volunteers involved. Although team spirit exists in acute care as well, there is often little time during work to provide each other support to enhance that spirit. Financial cutbacks threaten to reduce the amount of time that hospice care teams can provide mutual support as well.

- There is more open and honest communication between caregivers and the patient and family which decreases the likelihood that different caregivers will not share some of the information they have.
- There is great patient/family satisfaction and approval of hospice care teams that reflects well on the caregivers. In the home, hospice care teams have been invited in to help which adds a special dimension of intimacy and satisfaction.
- There is often specialized training for hospice caregivers which prepares them for their work. Part of this training is recognizing the cultural and religious diversity of people in North America. We cannot expect a first generation Chinese person to have the same general attitudes toward dying, death and bereavement as a fourth-generation Canadian with Italian and Scottish roots.
- There are fewer unpredictable situations as many terminal illnesses have a relatively well understand process toward a natural death. Symptoms may still change quickly, however, hospice care teams can help prepare patients and families for what is likely to happen in the months ahead.

Hospice care offers people an opportunity, every day, to make a dramatic and measurable difference in someone's life. What an opportunity to fulfill one of our greatest needs – to feel needed and to know that our life has meaning.

SUPPORTING OUR FRIENDS WHO ARE CAREGIVERS

The older we get the more likely we become caregivers for others. We can also help our friends when they are providing a lot of care to a loved one. In return, one day, these friends can provide us with similar supports when we need it most.

Here is a short list of things you can do to help. Keep in mind that you can adapt many of the suggestions to your particular situation.

- Be there. Be physically present as often as you can without intruding on your friends need to be alone with their loved one.
- Tell the person that they can call you in the middle of the night if they need some reassurance, encouragement or specific information they know you have. This offer will be used rarely but

just knowing there are people out there who can help in the middle of the night is very reassuring.

- Provide whatever stability you can by doing things on a schedule. This gives your friend something to look forward too. "It's Tuesday today. That means Sue is coming over this afternoon for a visit!"
- Help the person know that they cannot plan weeks ahead because they won't know how the illness will progress. There are certainly trends in the progress of people who have specific conditions but there are lots of variables.

  Therefore, encourage them to take each day as a miracle of time and loving with the person they love. Help them to adapt to changing circumstances. Help them to see what is special about this day.
- Take the person away for short walks, a snack, a movie, shopping, dining, etc. They may not want to leave their loved one so respect that. If another family member or friend can be there with the person who is ill, perhaps your friend will feel more comfortable in getting out for a bit.
- Understand the caregivers need laughter, love

and tears like everyone else. Don't presume to know what they need. Ask them.

- Provide information that will be helpful now or later on. People often have concerns or worries late at night and will pick up some information you have provided them that they find helpful.
- Invite your friend over for tea or a meal. People often don't eat as well when they are providing care for someone. Give them a nutritious, tasty meal and provide them with the leftovers to take home.
- Make frozen meals to bring over so they don't have to cook. Or bring over a fresh fruit or garden salad with a specialty dressing to make it extra special.
- Send or bring over fresh supplies of fruits, healthy treats, ice creams and such.
- If you are farther away call regularly and send cards, emails, notes, letters, music CDs, movies on DVD, etc. Stay in touch in this way so the person knows you are thinking of them. They may not read everything, watch everything or listen to everything, but they will know they are loved.

HOW CHILDREN AND TEENAGERS CAN HELP

Many parents presume that their younger children and teenagers should not be involved in providing physical, emotional, spiritual or information supports to loved ones. They think the children will either not want to or the parents may think they are protecting their children from some of the unpleasantness of providing care.

Many of today's boomer generation and their children have little or no experience caring for loved ones at home. I certainly did not. We were prevented, "for our own good," from participating in this kind of care. The result is that many of us are afraid to even try and learn and benefit from providing care.

Care has many life-affirming and life-defining opportunities built into it. Some of your fondest memories of loved ones may be of times you cared for them. Some of your greatest accomplishments will be those times when you helped someone live at home during their recovery, illness or death.

Children and teenagers should not be prevented from experiencing some of these same joys.

Young children and teenagers can be asked

what kind of help they would like to provide at home. They might help someone with their errands, answer some mail for them, read to them in bed, or make sure that neighbors and friends can come and visit. They may also be encouraged to watch as you provide physical care. They can be asked what things they might be interested in learning, such as feeding, bathing, or turning the person in bed.

They may help getting their loved one to the bedroom or bathroom.

There are some aspects of care that may be more unpleasant for some people than for others. These may include odors, unfamiliar degrees of intimacy, and cleaning up after the person. Others may be more disturbed by new expectations of helping that will reduce their time spent with friends.

Older children and teenagers may also have a heightened awareness of their own body and, therefore, may be more uncomfortable providing intimate personal care when helping their loved one. Recognizing these possible areas of discomfort make it possible for you to openly discuss everyone's concerns.

In this way each individual can list those aspects

of care they are most comfortable in providing and which they would prefer, if possible, that someone else do. For example, I was uncomfortable giving my mother a full-body bed bath. My father recognized this and did that part of her care. I was able to stay up throughout the night to provide support and care to my mother so that my father could get a relatively good night sleep before work the next day. We helped each other while helping my mother.

There are times, however, when one cannot pick and choose what they must do. Many of life's events have similar unpleasantness–few of us, for example, enjoyed studying for exams, taking out the garbage or being involved in the annual spring cleaning. But even during these times, we have fond memories of studying with someone we liked very much, playing with the dog as we took the garbage out or dumping all the dirty clothes over someone's head during spring cleaning. Caring for loved ones has similar opportunities for humor, laughter and play while the serious work gets done as well. Caring for loved ones also has profound moments of awareness, thoughtfulness, intimacy and love.

These should not be missed.

CARING FROM A DISTANCE

There are very practical things you can do to help from a distance. Much of what you do depends on whether there are family and friends nearby who can help your loved one when you cannot.

When There are Family and Friends to Help

Most of this section assumes that you are the main caregiver who is coordinating care, as best as possible, from a distance. However, if there are local family members and friends able to provide care and coordination, your role might be quite different.

The person farthest away often feels quite isolated from the day-to-day activities around their loved one's care. At the same time, the ones close by are often overwhelmed with juggling care of the loved one with all of their other commitments (e.g., to their own growing family, to their work and community commitments). In such situations there is less time for ongoing communication and that can lead to friction.

Having been on both sides of this equation, I know how important it is that everyone recognizes the stresses of the other person as best they can.

With you being far from your loved one, your contribution can be making regular phone calls or communication through e-mail, letters, flowers, and cards. As well, you can provide encouragement and support to those providing the day-to-day care. They need to know that you are thinking of them and not just leaving them to do all of the thinking and support.

Your ability to listen to their stories of joy and frustration can be very helpful. As well, since you are farther away you are likely working or, at least, not loosing part of your funds in providing day-to-day support. You could offer those providing care some extra money to allow them some much needed respite care (e.g., a weekly massage, a weekend away from home which would require some paid nursing care perhaps).

At the same time, your long distance suggestions cannot be based solely on what you would do if you were there because you are not. The people there need to be allowed to do the best they can given their circumstances.

You might wish that someone was there more often, or helped more with meal preparation or supported to visit friends. You cannot 'coach' from a distance without creating a great deal of tension.

The people providing care also know that their loved one often 'lights up' when you call. That is only natural as you are far away and, therefore, your call is special. However, it is important to recognize that your family members and friends providing the care also need your 'special' calls of encouragement and support.

At a distance you can volunteer to do some of the telephoning of others farther away so that those providing the day-to-day care do not have to do all the phoning. You can also help with 'paper-work' chores like some of the legal, financial, and if needed, funeral preparations. You can help by getting the basic information that those close by need to make decisions.

There may also be a need to do some library or Internet research about your loved one's condition and treatment that those nearby cannot find the time to do. Do not overwhelm them with information but rather provide them with some concise information they can use in talking to the decision makers about next steps. This can be an invaluable gift you provide your loved ones and those caring for them.

For those close by, especially in situations where a loved one's health is at great risk, please understand that everyone far away listens to each telephone ring as the one that leads to a call with bad news 'from home'. Recognize that being far away is isolating and lonely. Circumstances prevent those far away from being at the loved one's bedside and that is hard.

This mutual understanding is what makes it possible to be supportive from far away. Talk as often as possible and exchange thoughts and feelings to be supportive of each other and, therefore, supportive of the person requiring the home care.

When There are No Family or Friends to Help

When there are no family members or friends nearby to provide support, you must look at other alternatives. Depending on your loved one's needs and financial circumstances, you may need to ensure they stay in hospital or a rehabilitation center a bit longer, if possible, as there will not be enough home supports. Even with home care services provided through government and private organizations, there may be several days where

it would be unsafe to go home. This is where assertive advocacy may be necessary. You will need to have the telephone numbers of the decision makers in the hospital or center to ensure that you can get to them before your loved one is discharged.

Once at home, and depending on your loved one's need for help, a daily check-in call by you or a visit by a paid professional/volunteer may be the least that needs to be done to ensure your loved one's safety and that they know they are not alone as they recover from surgery or illness.

If you have time to prepare in advance, you can check with the local home care services offered by the government or for-profit organizations.

If you do not have time before a medical emergency to arrange that, you will need to contact the hospital or rehabilitation center's discharge planner even sooner to help ensure the person is seen everyday once they return home.

It is easy to say you should plan for these situations in advance. However, that is difficult to do given all the demands on your time. If you are reading this book because of a medical emergency, concentrate on the short-term things that need to get done. Use this opportunity to learn what you can do about longer range planning after this event is over.

Note: The following information assumes you cannot be with your loved one quickly.

Short-Term Situations

Short-term situations are often about 'crisis management' and so you will be tired and frustrated that you cannot do more or that you cannot get everything for your loved one when they need it. It is not comforting to know that this situation may be a bit like 'just getting through it is okay' but that might be the best that is possible for now. Once you have a bit more time and more information upon which to make decisions with your loved one, it will all feel more comfortable and do-able.

- Your greatest opportunity in the short term is to act as an assertive advocate for your loved one.

Firmly and fairly talk to the decision makers about what has happened, what needs to happen next and what must be in place before the person goes home.

- Next, you need to ensure that your loved one has access to a telephone, if they are able to speak. You want to be in contact as much as you can given their circumstance and your own.
- If they need to stay at the hospital or rehabilitation centre for more than a few days, see if there are any volunteers, social workers, or pastoral care workers who can come and spend some time with your loved one and who can contact you with any news, questions or concerns.
- Telephone and e-mail are both excellent tools to keep in touch with busy people.
- If the short-term situation will take a matter of days, see if you can get time away from work and/or home commitments to concentrate on getting what is needed for your loved one. If you can actually go and visit them during this situation, that would be great. Given that is not possible in many situations, you will need to ask for the help of your own family and friends nearby

to ensure you have the time and information you need to be as helpful as possible to your loved one. Telephone calling and e-mails have inevitable frustrating aspects to them. You will not always get to the right person at the right time which means you need extra time to make those contacts.

Long-Term Situations

When you have more time to plan, you gain a sense of comfort and control when you plan in advance. This planning may be necessary because your loved one is going in for surgery in a few months or because they need ongoing, long-term help because of disability or aging.

Although it is said elsewhere in this book, you need to take care of yourself in long-term care situations, even when you are far away. It is too easy to get caught up in the telephone calls, e-mails and research. You need to include those who love you, who live with you and live nearby. You need physical, emotional, spiritual and information supports as much as your loved one.

Ensure that you get it. Care giving is mutual

and you need to ask for help before your own health is hurt.

Whatever time you have to prepare, here are some tips to help you gain as much control over the situation as possible:

- In the *Caring for Loved Ones at Home* is a chapter on "Creating Your Own Support Team." It is full of information that can help you and your loved one feel a sense of control over future events. Creating a support team may require you to visit your loved one and use some of that time to plan together whom to ask to be part of such a team. Neighbors can be wonderfully helpful when asked to do specific things. Colleagues from your loved one's work, members of their spiritual community, and members from any organizations or community groups they belong to can be a rich source of participants in such a team. Your first goal is to find someone who will act as a coordinator of a team and the person who will keep in touch with you most often.
- Do not underestimate how many people may be willing to help. The key is knowing how to ask.

For example, which of the following requests for help from a neighbor would you be most likely to accept:

- "My Mom is pretty sick. Can you help us?" versus "My Mom is pretty sick. We were wondering if you might be able to help by cooking a casserole for her once every two weeks or picking up her medications at the pharmacy every three weeks or so? Would you be able to do one of those two things for us?" The second request is specific and time limited. People know what you are asking for and can easily tell you honestly if they can help or not. The first request is too vague and will scare people. They may think you want them to spend many hours doing things they feel unqualified to do.
- Whether your loved one is a member of a specific faith community or not, such a community can be wonderfully helpful. The hospital pastoral care department or the faith community closest to your loved one's home are two excellent places to start. There is a growing movement to encourage faith communities to go back to their caregiving roots and your loved one can help

them achieve just that. Be diligent in finding the right group for your loved one.

- Check out local libraries, newspapers and voluntary organizations to see what the local community already offers that might help your loved one. Some of this can be done by Internet and telephone. Perhaps there is a seniors' center, a volunteer group, or a spiritual community that are already in place and ready to help. Your loved one may also be part of a close-knit group (e.g., art guild, bridge club) whose members would enjoy helping out.
- You will also need to get some paperwork in order. Some of this can be done during a visit with your loved one while some can be done from a distance. For example, your loved one should have Powers of Attorney for personal care and another for financial decisions. You may be their power of attorney for both as the loved one accepting responsibility for their care. You need to ensure that the family physician, specialists and hospital have that power of attorney on record.
- You will need to make a contact list of the family physician, specialists, lawyer, accountant, funeral

home directors and others and contact them by phone or letter to let them know you will be coordinating care when your loved one is no longer able to do that for themselves.

- You will need to know where documents are kept and get some of them up-to-date, if necessary (e.g., Powers of Attorney, Last Will and Testament, marriage license, military papers, bank statements, other legal, financial, investment, and funeral pre-planning documents).
- Record all important information: social insurance numbers, health numbers, insurance policies, driver's licenses, credit cards, pre-planned funeral and internment information, passports, medications, emergency contact numbers (family physician, specialists, hospital, ambulance) as well as contact information for local friends of your loved one who can be called for help, if necessary.
- You will need to have information on all the utilities and other regular bills that come into the house in case you need to take over the handling of these bills.
- You will want a copy of the home key. If your

loved one agrees, you may also find it helpful to have copies of other important keys (e.g., car, cottage, safety deposit boxes) or know where they are kept. See if your loved one will also give a home key to a trusted neighbor in cases of emergency and give you their phone numbers. You may also consider a home monitoring system so that your loved one can call for help without using a telephone.

- It might help to have contact information for local basic home repair companies to respond to any emergency repairs (e.g., flooding toilet or basement drain, a broken furnace).
- You will need to let your family and employer know that you may be called away suddenly to care for a loved one for a while. Your work needs to be organized in such a way that someone can fill in for you without too much inconvenience for them or your employer. For example, if you are in an administrative role at work, you might have a binder filled with what you do, how you process things and get the work done. Someone who fills in for you during vacations or medical emergencies would be very pleased to have that.

- There may be a time when you need to go to your loved one to handle their transition from hospital or rehabilitation center back home. Again, knowing this is possible allows you to prepare for it. If it is not a complete surprise to family, friends and your work, then it is more likely you will get the support you need.
- It can be helpful to have a separate savings account, travel miles or credit card for emergency trips to loved ones. These trips will happen one day and if there is no financial difficulty in going to a loved one, it is one less stress you have to deal with.
- Check with your employer and government to see if they have any compassionate leave policies that would allow you to take time from work to care for your loved one. In the extreme case of your loved one dying, your employer or government may have a leave through their unemployment insurance plan to help cover some of your income loss during this time. Checking in advance about such policies can ease your mind a bit.

We have all been, and will all be, caregivers. If you have an elderly parent, you will likely be involved in caregiving. If you have young children, you will be involved in caregiving when they have an accident or a sickness.

These are predictable events – we just don't know when they will happen.

Just as with anything worthwhile in life, a bit of planning up front saves a lot of stress and problems later on. It is why we learn about our finances. It is why we read articles about improving our health. It should also be why, we take some time with family and friends to think about how we will deal with the next caregiving situation we are predictably going to be have. We will either be helping a family member or friend deal with their caregiving situation or they will be helping us.

A bit of planning means that we can actually enjoy much of the caregiving experience. It offers us so many opportunities to talk, laugh, share thoughts and experiences. Rather than being a frightening or disruptive experience, caregiving can be one of life's gifts that allow us to think, talk, plan and practice what we are going to do with the rest of our life.

Enjoy it all.

CHAPTER 8

Professional, Volunteer and Systemic Tips

Once a year I suggest you either: become a patient, follow a patient through the system, answer the telephones at a health care facility and/or shadow a front-line health-care worker for a while. This will help you practice, model and teach some of the following ideas and to experience the perspective of patients and their families. Walking with a patient and their family through a part of their process is the single best way to understand how everything you do impacts the patient and family.

Caution: Family caregivers must be seen and respected as children, spouses, parents, friends and neighbors **first and foremost**. We need to label them as family caregivers in discussions about their role in care, but we should never presume that caregiving is how they identify themselves. They are more likely to self-identify based on their relationship with the person who is ill rather than in their role of caring for that person.

The following are a list of ideas to help you in your professional and volunteer work. Some are specific ideas you can do without having to get permission from your program or service. Others will require you to work with your colleagues to enhance your program and service to better meet the physical, emotional, spiritual and information needs your patients and their families.

1. **Value the life of patients.** To provide excellent care you must begin with the belief that their life is worth living. The phrase we looked at earlier in this book – "I would rather be dead than..." – prevents you from seeing a person's life as worth living if you believe you would rather be dead than have a similar condition. You need to identify those conditions and come up with a thoughtful response of how you value the life of that specific patient or transfer your work over to someone else who

can.

2. **Value and enhance the social roles of patients.** People receive the best care possible when those around them see them in valued social roles like their role as parent, spouse, worker, volunteer, community leader, teacher, etc. Even when the person can no longer fulfill their role because of their illness, any new staff and volunteers working with that person needs to be told about all the valued roles this person played. It is not hard to believe that a much loved parent and community leader would get better care than a person without family nearby whose past history is little known or understood. You can help every patient identify their valued social roles and help others recognize those valued qualities in the person they are caring for.
3. **It is relatively easier for smaller programs and organizations to be patient-centered.** If you cannot be small, learn from those that are. Learn from those who practice closest to their community members rather than in departments in large

institutions. Learn how to move from identifying patients by numbers or conditions and truly see the person receiving care. Understand that smaller program staff has more opportunities to get to know each other's strengths and weaknesses and, therefore, build a stronger team of care providers. Learn how publicity, fundraising, accounting and community awareness of the programs are all different when done in small, accountable and well run programs.

4. **Minimize the number of people involved in caring for each patient.** It is true that this may difficult to schedule and more costly (from an organization's perspective versus the incalculable cost to patients and families) but it is one of the most critical aspects of systemic care today. At the end of one's life, you want to minimize as much as possible new people entering their lives. Not only does this mean yet one more person for the patient to get to know but they also become one more person to whom they have to say goodbye. Any changes in staffing or volunteers also requires more patient and family "training" of the new

person to get them to understand the person's medical history and current needs and hopes for end-of-life care. Each time the stories must be repeated is time taken away from caring for the person and the family. Time is obviously precious and should not be wasted on 'training' new staff or volunteers.

5. **Well-trained staff must understand, practice and model excellent physical, emotional, spiritual and information care**. It is not enough to acquire knowledge and skills. Many health care providers know how to provide excellent care but are discouraged by time and resource restraints from providing that care. They may also be restrained by untrained colleagues (whether in their own discipline or from another one) who do not want anyone else telling them how to provide better care. These are internal, communication and training issues that need immediate address. By law health care providers must report suspected cases of child or elder abuse. Ethically, one must also ensure that patients receive excellent palliative care. Anything less

is often tortuous and abusive – it is why, after all, the hospice movement was started.

6. **End turf wars.** Show the leadership that patients expect, need and demand to work together cooperatively. Do not make the patient or their loved ones suffer for systemic difficulties. Speak up on their behalf to regulators, governments and funders. That someone in one part of a city or community receives better care because their program got funding while another did not, is unacceptable. That one's care is more dependent on how powerful their care providers are relative to others is unacceptable. That care providers will actually fight for resources and money without regard to the effects on patients and their families (the 'empire builders') is unacceptable. We must start by examining the results of our 'turf' wars on patients and their families. Then we can better deal with negotiating equity division of limited resources.
7. **Advocate for equitable pay scales** between institutional and community care (e.g., in some towns and cities, community

nurses receive about 50% of what hospital nurses earn without benefits or job security). This is just wrong. Care in the community is not easier, nor less important. Nurses should not have to decide on the kind of nursing they want to do solely on where they can earn the most money. More and more patients are receiving care at home and deserve qualified, committed nurses to provide the care. There should be no second-class professionals providing care at home. They all deserve equal compensation based on their knowledge and skills, not where they practice.

8. **Recruit a broader range of staffing** so that one or two cultural groups do not represent the majority of your staff (especially in diverse multicultural communities). When we travel abroad, we often gravitate to people from "back home." This is natural. At the end of life, many people return to speaking their mother language and remembering their youth. The more diverse our working force, the more we can help people emotionally as well as physically and spiritually.

9. **Replace some of the high-tech, costly and ineffective treatments for a more humane, holistic care**. For cancer patients, as an example, 75% of all the health care money spent in your life from the moment of conception to death, is spent is the last year of your life – and they die anyway. Surely we can reallocate dollars so that excellent physical, emotional, spiritual and information needs are met without costly, intrusive, tortuous treatments that do not improve someone's last months of life.
10. Follow the age-old wisdom of ancient religions (and health care systems): **do unto others.** Build the type of care programs that you will want to use one day for your families and for yourself. All of the excuses used not to provide excellent care mean absolutely nothing to people who need that care. It will be the same for you and your family. Arguments against consistent staffing, limited resources, turf wars are all things that matter to people who run and work in systems, but not the end users and recipients of the system. Concentrate on

results rather than on processes to provide the greatest impact for everyone involved.

11. **Many vulnerable patients are voiceless in our health care system. Advocate strongly on their behalf.** Put the emphasis on patients with long-term care needs, our frail elders, people with disabilities, our patients needing palliative care and our fellow citizens who are poor who have few outside resources. These non-vocal and mostly non-voting family, friends and neighbors should not continue to be the victims of systemic problems. We must stop inflicting harm on those of us who are already harmed so much by their devalued status in our communities.

Our expectations must be based on an understood, practiced, disseminated and monitored philosophy of patient care that includes everyone having access to effective physical, emotional, spiritual and informational supports to live fully until their deaths. Their families, friends and care providers need to receive similar support and after-death bereavement supports if necessary. A person's background (age, gender, income level, language, education, etc.) cannot be a determining factor. We have enough examples of excellent care now to know what it should look like. The challenge is to replicate consistently and predictably what we know works well.

CHAPTER 9

Community Action The Goal of a Pain-Free Community

If we are going to have the type of care we want for our own loved ones, and for ourselves, then we must change the systems of care available now. We begin with the undeniable fact that:

No one who is dying needs to have unbearable pain – no one.

To experience it, unrelieved, is negligent and immoral.

We must recognize that:

- 75% of all health care money spent in a life time for cancer patients is spent in our last year and they die anyway (therefore, reallocate funding to include more for home care, palliative care),

- we have the knowledge, skills and resources now to provide excellent care,
- we must support hospice care providers more effectively,
- we must co-ordinate effective care locally,
- we must limit the growth of individual hospice care services (small is better than big),
- we must limit government funding and return to endowment funds, donations and workers (professional and volunteer) who see hospice work as a vocation rather than a career.
- No one who is dying needs to have unbearable pain – no one. To experience it, unrelieved, is negligent and immoral.

In a bilingual survey Legacies commissioned in 2000 we found out that about 25,000 Canadians die each year with unbearable pain. This result was not based on a worst-case scenario. Rather the question we asked was **"When your loved one's pain was best managed, what was it on a scale of 1-10 with ten being the worst pain?"** Based on that question, about 25,000 Canadians each year have pain between 7-10, **when it was best**

managed!

Specifically the results by (Dialogue Canada), May 2000 (2,404 surveys returned) were:

- 1/3 adult Canadians had family member or close friend die of a terminal or life-threatening illness within previous 2 years
- 29% had pain that was **unsuccessfully** treated **most, or all, of the time**
- 28% had pain that was **unsuccessfully** treated **some of the time**
- when pain was most effectively controlled, 44% of these patients had terrible pain (between 7-10 on 10-point scale with 10 = very great pain) or approximately 25,000 per year.

We concluded that:

- There is no strong advocacy voice for patients (although many agencies, services, organizations and associations represent professionals and volunteer care providers).
- Too few people receive any form of effective palliative care (physical, emotional, spiritual, information).

- Insufficient leadership within health care and insufficient political will to resolve these obvious problems quickly and effectively.
- Insufficient thoughtfulness on preventing a repeat of modern health care bureaucratization and expansion; and short-term view of integrating into ineffective system.

HOW HAVE THINGS IMPROVED?

Advocacy for patients is increasing. The emphasis is still on systemic changes rather than patient-centered care with a strong family focus within a strong community orientation. We need more services loyal to the patient rather than to a system or funder.

The number of people receiving formal and informal palliative care has increased. Informal palliative care, well delivered, is better than formal because it involves people providing care that the patient already knows. The fewer new care providers in someone's life, the better.

Some of these programs have strayed from providing excellent physical, emotional, spiritual and information care. Some of becoming too large and too restricted in their ability to provide the patient-centered philosophy of palliative care.

A return to the philosophy as practiced in the 1970s and 1980s is necessary so that systems do not override individual patient needs. Large medical programs must not take over palliative care programs. The reverse is necessary. The philosophy of palliative care is the model for all medical and health care; namely, meeting a patient's physical, emotional, spiritual and information needs. You should not have to be dying to get this level of patient-centered care.

Pain and symptoms can always be helped so that people can live as fully as possible and participate in their family and community life.

Locally, you and your allies in the promotion of excellent hospice palliative care can:

1. require palliative/hospice care providers to demand of their colleagues in other branches of medicine, nursing, and social work to use the proven methods to control unbearable physical pain. We have legislated that care providers

must report child and elder abuse done by their colleagues; we can do the same to prevent the torturous neglect of dying people.

2. recognize pain as the fifth vital sign that must be monitored and addressed regularly by physicians and nurses (the other four being temperature, pulse, respiration and blood pressure). It is not acceptable to ignore pain and discomforting symptoms when we have the skills to control them.
3. educate the general public to understand and accept the basic principles of effective pain and symptom control so that they do not expect or accept, inadequate control of unbearable pain.
4. require health care administrators, insurance companies, and health care bureaucrats to ensure and monitor effective pain and symptom control and that they publicly and forcefully deal with those who negligently do not practice it.
5. demand legislators to revise laws and regulations to strongly encourage and monitor effective pain and symptom control and forcefully deal with those who negligently do not

practice it while safeguarding those who practice effective pain and symptom control from malicious prosecution.

If we do these things together, then when someone we know is dying, they will not suffer unbearable pain BUT RATHER be relatively pain-free and alert with the energy to live life to the fullest with their family and friends. We promote excellent hospice palliative care to improve the care of all community members but we also do it to ensure that our own families, and one day us, also have compassionate, personal care. This humane motive includes everyone we know and love as well as people we will never know. That is the hospice palliative care philosophy represented at its best and we control the outcomes when we work together.

CHAPTER 10

Pulling It Together

How do we apply what we have learned? First you concentrate on what is actually possible for you to do and do those things in positive ways.

In other words, you cannot individually change the systems of care to ensure that each of your patients and their families has excellent care. You need to concentrate on what is possible within your authority and work on those aspects of care as best you can. Always begin with the person and their family.

Consider working with others to make systemic changes. Just as maternal care became more personalized and less technological when women in the community changed the thinking of medical providers, you can make changes within your community both at work and as a health care consumer.

All of us will die so this is one of the few health care issues that will touch every single one of us.

What you don't understand, let others teach you. None of us can know everything about providing excellent care in all situations with all people. Find those people who can teach you and learn from them. Then pass it on. What you know well, teach and role model to others.

We only change our behavior when we hold ourselves accountable. So:

1. What one or two things can you do differently after today?
2. What one or two thing can you do more often?
3. How can you help/teach even more than you do now?
4. Who is your role model for providing excellent care?
5. Are you someone's role model? How can you help/teach them even more?

The greatest motivator in the world is to feel useful and appreciated. Recognize that each day of your personal and professional life, you can make a significant and life-affirming difference in other people's lives and, therefore, a difference in your own life. These are mutual gifts we can offer and accept. Few things will have as profound impact on your personal life and the life of your community.

References

CHPCA April 10, 2006 Monthly Update e-newsletter and May 2006 Fact Sheet of CHPCA statistics at

http://www.chpca.net/events/nhpc_week/2006/Factsheet-HospicePalliativeCarein Canada-May2006.pdf for most current statistics.

Dass, Ram and Gorman, Paul. (1987). *How can I help?: Stories and reflections on service.* New York: Alfred A. Knopf.

Expert Advisory Committee on the Management of Severe Chronic Pain in Cancer Patients. (1984, 1987). *Cancer pain: A monograph on the management of cancer pain.* Ottawa: Ministry of Supply and Services. Excellent summary of modern pain control techniques; distributed to all Canadian physicians.

Hospice Journal, 1995, Vol 10, #1 pages 1-13.

Ley, Dorothy C.H. with Harry van Bommel. (1994). *The heart of hospice*. Toronto: NC Press, dedication page.

Parliamentary Committee on Palliative and Compassionate Care. (Nov 2011). *Not to be forgotten: Care of vulnerable Canadians.* http://pcpcc-cpspsc.com/wp-content/uploads/2011/11/ReportEN.pdf (accessed January 20, 2012)

van Bommel, Harry. (2006). *Caring for loved ones at home*. Toronto: Legacies Inc.

van Bommel, Harry. (2006). *Family hospice care: Pre-planning and care guide*. Toronto: Legacies Inc.

THE WORLD WIDE WEB (INTERNET)

The following Internet links may be helpful for people interested in more information about hospice/palliative and home care. I have picked just a few sites that have excellent resources and extensive links to other related sites. These organizations deserve a lot of credit for the effort they have put into their Web sites.

***A note of caution**: There are thousands of Web sites offering health care information. The information on some sites may not be accurate or current. Check to see who produces the Web site, their qualifications and their credibility before assuming their information is correct.*

Also, when checking the Web or other sources, for health care information, expect to find information that might be unsettling. The information may tell you things you didn't expect or didn't want to know and it may have been written for a professional audience rather than for patients and families.

Our own web sites has many free online resources available to the readers. Visit www.legacies.ca, www.carelibrary.com, and www.navcare.org to find resources on all aspects of health and hospice palliative care.

For general health information, **Health Canada's Information Site**: *www.hc-sc.gc.ca*

An extensive site with many links to other reputable sites.

Canadian Health Network

www.canadian-health-network.ca

A general health information site with links to many other health related sites.

The Association for Death Education and Counseling *www.adec.org* and the **King's College Centre for Education about Death and Bereavement** *www.deathed.ca* are useful sites for those interested in teaching or learning more about death, dying and bereavement.

Centre for Disease Control and Prevention

http://www.cdc.gov/omhd

Dr. Koop's Community

www.drkoop.com

An interactive health site with daily updates and news. Dr. Koop was for the former U.S. Surgeon General.

The Institute of Palliative Care in Ottawa has an extensive links section to organizations around the country and globe *www.pallcare.org/links.htm* Their whole site is worth a visit.

Mayo Clinic.Com

www.mayoclinic.com

An outstanding site for general health information

The **National Hospice Palliative Care Organization** in the U.S. *www.nhpco.org* provides many links to hospice programs throughout America and other organizations.

Hospice Association of Ontario Lifeline (Toronto) has many sources and links at *www.hospicelifeline.com*

Results Not Intentions is a Legacies Inc. website to highlight professional research on the inequality of patient care and how we might address those inequalities to ensure excellent care for everyone.

www.resultsnotintentions.com

UpToDate

www.uptodate.com

A clinical reference for physicians who subscribe but also includes patient information that is updated regularly.

The **World Health Organization** is another extensive site for health related information *http://www.who.int/*

What HOSPICE CARE Means to Me

Nurture relationships above all else.

Heal my wounds during my tests, treatments, and diagnosis so I can live fully until I die

Organize care of my family and me so we are seen as whole, as we are, rather than diseased, or as systemic 'units of care'

Spiritual care sees us all as children of God or nature rather than as patients and caregivers

Physical care takes away my pain and suffering while providing comfort and support

Information care helps me understand my options

Compassion is "walking with me" and being present in the moment

Emotional care supports my living on a roller coaster of feelings and thoughts

Communicate with me (not at me) and my family in a "common" language of understanding
Aggressive palliative supports so that I can concentrate on my family and friends
Responsibly concentrate on your part of my care and advocate for me with others
Eternal consequences of your care affects you and me forever.

Thank you!

Index